Mit den besten Empfehlungen

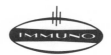

Immuno GmbH · Slevogtstraße 3–5 · 6900 Heidelberg 1

Fibrinklebung mit Tissucol®

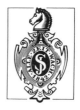

G. Schlag H. Redl (Eds.)

Fibrin Sealant
in Operative Medicine

Volume 7

Traumatology – Orthopaedics

Springer-Verlag
Berlin Heidelberg New York
London Paris Tokyo

Professor Dr. Günther Schlag
Dozent Dipl.-Ing. Dr. Heinz Redl
Ludwig-Boltzmann-Institut
für experimentelle Traumatologie
Donaueschingenstraße 13
A-1200 Vienna

Tissucol or Tisseel are registered trademarks of IMMUNO's two-component fibrin sealant in different countries

---

ISBN 3-540-17281-5 Springer-Verlag Berlin Heidelberg New York
ISBN 0-387-17281-5 Springer-Verlag New York Berlin Heidelberg

Printing: Beltz Offsetdruck, 6944 Hemsbach/Bergstraße
Bookbinding: J. Schäffer, 6718 Grünstadt

2127/3140-543210

Preface

Fibrin plays a prominent role in wound healing. It has a hemostatic effect, induces cellular response to wound damage, and, by forming strands to build a matrix, assists in neovascularization and fibroblast proliferation.

The concept of using clotting substances from human blood for wound management and to achieve hemostasis in bleeding parenchymatous organs can be traced to 1909, when Bergel [1] reported on the hemostatic effect of fibrin powder. In 1915, Grey [3] employed fibrin to control bleeding in neurosurgical operations of the brain. A year later, Harvey [4] used fibrin patches to stop bleeding from parenchymatous organs in general surgery.

It took more than two decades for this ingenious idea to be rediscovered. In 1940, Young and Medawar [8] reported on experimental nerve anastomosis by sealing. Similarly, Tarlov and Benjamin [7] reunited nerves with plasma clots in 1943. Tarlov improved the results obtained with clot anastomosing of nerves by avoiding tension at the nerve stumps. In 1944, Cronkite et al. [2] reported on an initial series of eight cases in which fibrinogen and thrombin had been used successfully for anchoring skin grafts.

Although these early attempts suggested the basic advantages of using a biomaterial for wound closure – such as complete absorption, improved wound healing, and excellent tissue tolerance – the failure rate was relatively high, mainly because the fibrinogen employed had poor adhesive strength and the sealing did not last. It was because of these unsatisfactory results that the technique was not further pursued in the decades to follow.

In 1972, the use of fibrin as a biologic adhesive was revived by Matras et al. [6], who successfully employed a fibrinogen cryoprecipitate for reuniting peripheral nerves in an animal model. Matras and Kuderna used autologous material in the first successful human application in 1975 [5]. It was not until a special cryoprecipitation process had been developed that it was possible to produce a highly concentrated fibrinogen solution with an enriched factor XIII content, as the basis of two-component fibrin sealant.

In the meantime, the controversial issue of virus transmission, including the transmission of HTLV-III, by the blood product Tisseel (Tissucol) has been resolved. In addition to subjecting Tisseel (Tissucol) to in-process virus inactivation, both the source material and final product are routinely screened for HTLV-III antibody.

Following the first international symposium on fibrin sealant in Vienna in 1985, which dealt with the use of the product in various surgical disciplines, this seven-volume study attempts to present current knowledge relating to the method of fibrin sealing. The disciplines covered are: general and abdominal surgery; ophthalmology and neurosurgery; otorhinolaryngology; plastic, maxillofacial and dental surgery; thoracic and cardiovascular surgery; traumatology and orthopaedics; urology, gynaecology and obstetrics. Each volume is preceded by a general chapter on the principles of fibrin sealing, methods of application, aspects of quality control, and safety studies.

Today, fibrin sealing has become an accepted tool in many fields of surgery. In many areas, fibrin sealing has superseded conventional surgical techniques, increased postoperative safety, and even made new therapeutic approaches possible.

We would like to thank all authors for their excellent contributions and helpful photographs, which have made these seven volumes on fibrin sealing possible.

Vienna, Juni 1986   G. Schlag
                                                                              H. Redl

Table of Contents

List of Contributors

I. Principles of Fibrin Sealing

BAUMGARTEN, K., Prof. Dr.
Geburtshilflich-gynäkologische Abteilung, Wilhelminen-Spital, Montleartstraße 37,
1160 Wien, Austria

CERWENKA, R., Dr.
Geburtshilflich-gynäkologische Abteilung, Wilhelminen-Spital, Montleartstraße 37,
1160 Wien, Austria

DINGES, H.P., Dr.
Institut für pathologische Anatomie, Universität Graz, Auenbruggerplatz 25,
8036 Graz, Austria

EDER, G., Dr.
Immuno AG, Clinical Research, Gastroenterology, Sandwirtgasse 3,
1060 Wien, Austria

NEUMANN, M., Dr.
Geburtshilflich-gynäkologische Abteilung, Wilhelminen-Spital, Montleartstraße 37,
1160 Wien, Austria

PFLÜGER, H., Doz.
Urologische Abteilung, Allgemeines österreichisches Krankenhaus,
Kremser Landstraße 36, 3100 St. Pölten, Austria

REDL, H., Doz.
Ludwig-Boltzmann-Institut für Experimentelle Traumatologie,
Donaueschingenstraße 13, 1200 Wien, Austria

SCHLAG, G., Prof. Dr.
Ludwig-Boltzmann-Institut für Experimentelle Traumatologie,
Donaueschingenstraße 13, 1200 Wien, Austria

TURNHER, M., Dr.
Ludwig-Boltzmann-Institut für Experimentelle Traumatologie,
Donaueschingenstraße 13, 1200 Wien, Austria

II. Traumatology

ANDREASSEN, T. T., Dr.
Department of Connective Tissue Biology, University of Aarhus, 4000 Aarhus C,
Denmark

ARZINGER-JONASCH, A., Prof. Dr.
Chirurgische Klinik, Karl-Marx-Universität, Liebigstraße 20 A, 7010 Leipzig,
German Democratic Republic

ANTONINI, C., Dr.
Institute of Emergency Surgery, Policlinic of Perugia, Via A. Brunamonti,
06100 Perugia, Italy

BERNETT, B., Prof. Dr.
Lehrstuhl für Sporttraumatologie, Technische Universität München,
Connollystraße 32, 8000 München 40, Federal Republic of Germany

BÜNGER, C., Dr.
Institute for Experimental Clinical Research, University of Aarhus, 8000 Aarhus C,
Denmark

CASTAGNOLI, G., Dr.
Institute of Emergency Surgery, Policlinic of Perugia, Via A. Brunamonti,
06100 Perugia, Italy

EGKHER, E., Dr.
II. Universitätsklinik für Unfallchirurgie, Spitalgasse 23, 1090 Wien, Austria

GAUDERNAK, T., Dr.
Lorenz-Böhler-Krankenhaus der Allgemeinen Unfallversicherungsanstalt,
Donaueschingenstraße 13, 1200 Wien, Austria

JØRGENSEN, P. H., Dr.
Department of Connective Tissue Biology, University of Aarhus, 8000 Aarhus C,
Denmark

JOYCE, F., Dr.
Institute of Experimental Clinical Research, University of Aarhus, 8000 Aarhus C,
Denmark

KEDRA, H., Dr.
Department of Experimental Surgery and Biomaterials Research, Clinic of Surgical
Traumatology, Medical Academy of Wroclaw, ul. Poniatowskiego 2,
50-326 Wroclaw, Poland

KELLER, J., Dr.
Institute of Experimental Clinical Research, University of Aarhus, 8000 Aarhus C, Denmark

KETTERL, R., Dr.
Chirurgische Klinik und Poliklinik rechts der Isar, Technische Universität München, Ismaninger Straße 22, 8000 München 80, Federal Republic of Germany

KNUDSEN, V. E., Dr.
Institute of Experimental Clinical Research, University of Aarhus, 8000 Aarhus C, Denmark

KRAKOVITS, G., Dr.
Department of Orthopaedic Surgery and Trauma János Kórhaz, Diósárok ut 1, 1125 Budapest, Hungary

KUS, H. Prof. Dr.
Clinic of Surgical Traumatology, Medical Academy of Wroclaw, ul. Traugutta 57/59, 50-417 Wroclaw, Poland

LANGE, R., Dr.
Chirurgische Klinik und Poliklinik rechts der Isar, Technische Universität München, Ismaninger Straße 22, 8000 München 80, Federal Republic of Germany

LUCHT, U., Dr.
Institute for Experimental Clinical Research, University of Aarhus, 8000 Aarhus C, Denmark

MERCATI, U., Prof. Dr.
Institute of Emergency Surgery, Policlinic of Perugia, Via A. Brunamonti, 06100 Perugia, Italy

MØLLER, J., Dr.
Institute for Experimental Clinical Research, University of Aarhus, 8000 Aarhus C Denmark

PAAR, O., Dr. Privatdozent
Lehrstuhl für Sporttraumatologie, Technische Universität München, Conollystraße 32, 8000 München 40, Federal Republic of Germany

PASSL, R., Doz. Dr.
Unfallchirurgische Abteilung, Krankenhaus der Barmherzigen Brüder, Esterhàzystraße 26, 7000 Eisenstadt, Austria

PLENK Jr, H., Prof. Dr.
Histologisch-Embryologisches Institut, Universität Wien, Schwarzspanierstraße 17, 1090 Wien, Austria

SANDNER, K.-H., Dr.
Chirurgische Klinik, Karl-Marx-Universität Leipzig, Liebigstraße 20 A,
7010 Leipzig, German Democratic Republic

SKORPIK, G., Dr.
Lorenz-Böhler-Krankenhaus der Allgemeinen Unfallversicherungsanstalt,
Donaueschingenstraße 13, 1200 Wien, Austria

SPÄNGLER, H., Prof. Dr.
II. Universitätsklinik für Unfallchirurgie, Spitalgasse 23, 1090 Wien, Austria

SPÄNGLER, H. P., Dr.
II. Universitätsklinik für Unfallchirurgie, Spitalgasse 23, 1090 Wien, Austria

STANISZEWSKA-KUS, J., Dr. biol.
Department for Experimental Surgery and Biomaterials Research, Clinic for
Surgical Traumatology, Medical Academy of Wroclaw, ul. Poniatowskiego 2,
50-326 Wroclaw, Poland

STÜBINGER, B., Privat-Dozent Dr.
Chirurgische Klinik und Poliklinik rechts der Isar, Technische Universität München,
Ismaninger Straße 22, 8000 München 80, Federal Republic of Germany

TACSIK, I., Dr.
Department of Orthopaedic Surgery and Trauma János Kórház, Diósárok ut 1,
1125 Budapest, Hungary

TILING, T., Privat-Dozent Dr.
Abteilung für Unfallchirurgie, II. Chirurgische Klinik, Universität Köln,
Ostmerheimer Straße 200, 5000 Köln 91, Federal Republic of Germany

ZIFKO, B., Dr.
Lorenz-Böhler-Krankenhaus der Allgemeinen Unfallversicherungsanstalt,
Donaueschingenstraße 13, 1200 Wien, Austria

ZILCH, H., Doz. Dr.
Orthopädische Klinik und Poliklinik, Freie Universität Berlin, Oskar-Helene-Heim,
Clayallee 229, 1000 Berlin 33, Federal Republic of Germany

III. Orthopaedics

ALBISETTI, W., Dr.
Istituto di Clinica Ortopedica, Universitá degli Studi Milano, Via Bignami 1,
20126 Milano, Italy

ARBES, H., Dr.
Orthopädisches Krankenhaus Gersthof, Wielemansgasse 28, 1180 Wien, Austria

ASCHERL, R., Dr.
Institut für Experimentelle Chirurgie, Technische Universität München,
Ismaninger Straße 13, 8000 München 80, Federal Republic of Germany

ATTOLINI, R., Dr.
Istituto di Clinica Ortopedica, University degli Studi Milano, Via Bignami 1,
20126 Milano, Italy

BAUDO, F., Dr.
Department of Haematology, Ospedale Niguarda-lá Granda, 20126 Milano, Italy

BECK, H., Prof. Dr.
Chirurgische Universitätsklinik Erlangen, Maximiliansplatz, 8520 Erlangen,
Federal Republic of Germany

BLÜMEL, G., Prof. Dr.
Institut für Experimentelle Chirurgie, Technische Universität München,
Ismaninger Straße 13, 8000 München 80, Federal Republic of Germany

BÖSCH, P., Doz. Dr.
Orthopädische Abteilung, Allgemeines Krankenhaus, Corvinusring 3–5,
2700 Wiener Neustadt, Austria

BONFIGLIO, G., Dr.
Istituto di Clinica Ortopedica II, Universitá degli Studi Milano, Via Bignami 1,
20126 Milano, Italy

BRAUN, A., Prof. Dr.
Septic Orthopedic Surgery Section, Orthopedics Division, University of Heidelberg,
Schlierbacher Landstraße 200a, 6900 Heidelberg, Federal Republic of Germany

de CATALDO, F., Dr.
Department of Haematology; Ospedale Niguarda-lá Granda, 20126 Milano, Italy

CEREA, P., Dr.
Istituto di Clinica Ortopedica, Universitá degli Studi Milano, Via Bignami 1,
20126 Milano, Italy

GEISSDÖRFER, K. Dr.
Institut für Experimentelle Chirurgie, Technische Universität München,
Ismaninger Straße 13, 8000 München 80, Federal Republic of Germany

GOUDARZI, Y. M., Privat-Dozent Dr.
Chirurgische Abteilung, Kinderklinik, Rudolf-Virchow-Krankenhaus,
Postfach 65 02 69, 1000 Berlin 65, Federal Republic of Germany

HERZOG, T., Dr.
Chirurgische Universitätsklinik Erlangen, Maximiliansplatz, 8520 Erlangen,
Federal Republic of Germany

KELLNER, G., Dr.
Universitätsklinik für Orthopädie, Garnisongasse 13, 9. Hof, 1090 Wien, Austria

LACK, W., Dr.
Universitätsklinik für Orthopädie, Garnisongasse 13, 9. Hof, 1090 Wien, Austria

LECHNER, F., Prof. Dr.
Krankenhaus Garmisch-Partenkirchen, 8100 Garmisch-Partenkirchen,
Federal Republic of Germany

LINTNER, F., Doz. Dr.
Institut für Pathologische Anatomie, Universität Wien, Spitalgasse 4, 1090 Wien,
Austria

LOZEJ, E., Dr.
Istituto di Clinica Ortopedica, Universitá degli Studi Milano, Via Bignami 1,
20126 Milano, Italy

MAPELLI, F., Dr.
Istituto di Clinica Ortopedica, Universitá degli Studi Milano, Via Bignami 1,
20126 Milano, Italy

MARINONI, E. C., Prof. Dr.
Istituto di Clinica Ortopedica II, Universitá degli Studi Milano, Via Bignami 1,
20126 Milano, Italy

MICALE, C., Dr.
Istituto di Clinica Ortopedica, Università degli Studi Milano, Via Bignami 1,
20126 Milano, Italy

MISTO, G., Dr.
Istituto di Clinica Ortopedica, Università degli Studi Milano, Via Bignami 1,
20126 Milano, Italy

MOINA, E. M., Dr.
Departamento de Traumatología y Cirugía Ortopédica Centro Especial "Ramón y
Cajal", Crtr. de Colmenar Km 9,100, 28034 – Madrid – Spain

MOLINARI, P., Dr.
Istituto di Clinica Ortopedica, Università degli Studi Milano, Via Bignami 1,
20126 Milano, Italy

PALACIOS-CARVAJAL, J., Dr. Prof.
Hospital Monografico Asepeyo de Traumatología, Cirugía Ortopédi ca y
Rehabilitación, C/. Joaquín de Cárdenas, 2 – Coslada (Madrid) – Spain

PALAZZI, F. F., Dr.
Cirurgia Ortopedica y Traumatologia, Apartado de Correos 66473,
Plaza Las Américas, Caracas 1061 A, Venezuela

POCHON, J.-P., Dr.
Chirurgische Abteilung, Kinderspital Zürich, Steinwiesstraße 75, 8032 Zürich,
Switzerland

RAMACH, W., Dr.
Universitätsklinik für Orthopädie, Garnisongasse 13, 9. Hof, 1090 Wien, Austria

RIVAS HERNANDEZ, S., Dr.
Cirurgia Ortopedica y Traumatologia, Apartado de Correos 66473,
Plaza Las Américas, Caracas 1061 A, Venezuela

RUPCICH, M., Dr.
Cirurgia Ortopedica y Traumatologia, Apartado de Correos 66473,
Plaza Las Américas, Caracas 1061 A, Venezuela

TORRI, G., Prof. Dr.
Istituto di Clinica Ortopedica, Università degli Studi Milano, Via Bignami 1,
20126 Milano, Italy

ULIVI, M., Dr.
Istituto di Clinica Ortopedica, Universitá degli Studi Milano, Via Bignami 1,
20126 Milano, Italy

WOLF, N., Dr. Dr. habil.
Chirurgische Universitätsklinik Erlangen, Maximiliansplatz, 8520 Erlangen,
Federal Republic of Germany

I. Principles of Fibrin Sealing

The Importance of Fibrin in Wound Repair

G. Schlag, H. Redl, M. Turnher, and H.P. Dinges

Key words: wound healing, fibrin, macrophages, granulocytes

Abstract

A review is given, beginning with the inflammatory phase of wound healing and explaining the role of macrophages, platelets, and granulocytes. Beside the cellular response the special importance of fibrin and factor XIII is demonstrated, particularly their function for fibroplasia. Special emphasis is put on the effect of highly concentrated fibrin – fibrin sealant. Its beneficial role in promoting the growth of fibroblasts is shown by a study on rats, in which a new model of granulation tissue formation was used. With this model it can be demonstrated that the application of fibrin sealant leads to significantly higher amounts of fibroblasts in newly formed granulation tissue. However, it is also demonstrated that fibrin sealant cannot overcome the inhibition of wound healing caused by, for example, adriamycin, though the beneficial effect of fibrin sealant in other cases of disturbed wound healing, e.g., ulcus cruris, has been demonstrated previously.

General Aspects

Three phases of wound healing are seen following trauma:
- Inflammatory phase
- Fibroplasia
- Protective maturation phase

Tissue trauma is immediately followed by coagulation and hemostasis. Coagulation eventually leads to conversion of fibrinogen into fibrin via the humoral pathway under the influence of thrombin and calcium (Fig. 1).

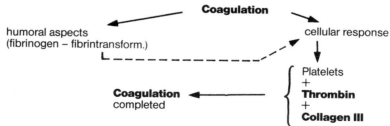

Fig. 1. Primary events following injury

Fibrin Sealant in Operative Medicine
Traumatology and Orthopaedics – Vol. 7
Edited by G. Schlag, H. Redl
© Springer-Verlag Berlin Heidelberg 1986

During the coagulation process, a cellular response is seen. Together with thrombin and collagen III, the platelets complete coagulation. Adhesion of the platelets to collagen fibrils of type III [3, 20] leads to platelet aggregation, where the platelets change from a reversible into an irreversible form. 5-Hydroxy-tryptamine and epinephrine are released from the platelets, which undergo further aggregation. Other substances are released from platelets, like platelet factor III, which acts on the formation of thrombin. Platelets are also important for the fibrin network structure, since they make fibrin more resistant to mechanical shear forces and to fibrinolysis [13].

The coagulation activated via humoral as well as cellular pathways leads to the blood clot which acts as a sealant primarily because of its fibrin content. In this way, normal hemostatic mechanisms help to prevent contamination and loss of body fluids as well as providing a substrate material for cell growth [2].

Fibrin is essential since it causes chemotaxis [24] of PMNs (in vitro) in the presence of fibrin degradation products. Fibrin mainly leads to recruitment in the injured tissue and also activates the macrophages.

Immediately after trauma and the ensuing coagulation, the inflammatory phase (lag phase) starts and extends to the 4th or 5th day. This phase is a vital part of the wound repair process. The local neutrophils (PMNs) increase within several hours. The main task of PMNs is to degrade damaged tissue (debriding) and to phagocytose cell debris. The migration of PMNs is presumably caused by chemotactic substances released from aggregated platelets or from plasma components (proteases, fibrinopeptide A). During the first 48 h the PMNs increase markedly and are quickly subject to lysis. Only a few are engaged in phagocytosis [22]. Evidence from studies using antineutrophil serum suggests that the PMNs are not essential in normal wound healing.

After some days, the most important cellular components in the inflammatory phase, i.e., the "monocytes", migrate (Fig. 2), change into macrophages, and reach their maximum number in the wound between the 4th and 5th day. The macrophages serve many different functions. According to Gustafson [15], these include regulation of coagulation (macrophage-induced procoagulant activity, factors V, VII, IX, and X) and fibrinolysis; elimination of cells, tissue debris, and bacteria; and regulation of fibroblast activity (fibroblast growth factor). Their main tasks include

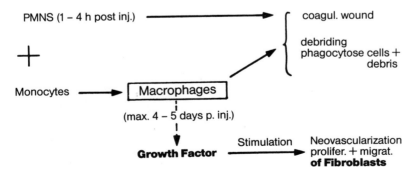

Fig. 2. Inflammatory phase of wound healing

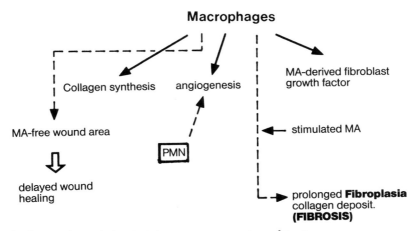

Fig. 3. The role of macrophages during the inflammatory phase of wound healing

phagocytosis of fibrin and the release of growth factors which stimulate fibroblast and endothelial cell proliferation in vitro [14, 28]. Induction of angiogenesis by wound macrophages has been confirmed [12, 21] (Fig. 3). Hunt et al [21] reported that this activity involved macrophages more than PMNs; however, a granulocyte component in the production of angiogenesis could not be excluded. Macrophages are responsible not only for neovascularization in the wound but also for stimulation of collagen synthesis. Collagen synthesis requires fibroplasia. Here, the "macrophage-derived fibroplast growth factor" apparently plays a vital part. If antimacrophage serum is administered, wound healing is severely delayed. On the other hand, prolonged activation of macrophages (endotoxin, bacterial products) may result in exaggerated fibroplasia and collagen deposition, which ends in fibrosis [21].

As to the cellular response in wound healing, the platelets in connection with fibrin play an important part [25]. Activated by thrombin, the platelets release a mitogen for fibroblasts and smooth muscle cells and stimulate collagen synthesis. This mitogen was isolated as "platelet-derived growth factor".

Fibroplasia and collagen synthesis start within 24 h following trauma. The platelets also activate neovascularization. Thus vital factors for wound healing are released by the platelets, which are largely responsible for the healing process (Fig. 4).

Wound healing is influenced by local oxygenation. Banda et al. [4] have shown that anoxia leads to stimulation and activation of the macrophages. This causes production of an angiogenesis factor and a macrophage-derived growth factor which stimulates the fibroblasts.

Knighton et al. [26] have demonstrated hypoxic stimulation of angiogenesis by macrophages in a corneal assay. Hyperoxia appears to suppress angiogenesis as shown in a second experiment with an ear chamber equipped with oxygen-perme-

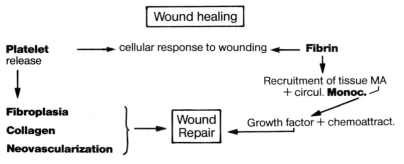

Fig. 4. The concert action of fibrin and platelets

able or -impermeable membranes. The demonstration that respiratory oxygen concentration affects the tensile strength of healing wounds and granulomas may reflect macrophage regulation of angiogenesis or fibroplasia [31, 32].

Granulation tissue plays a key role in the healing of all organs, except for those of epithelial origin. Granulation tissue largely consists of macrophages, endothelial cells, and fibroblasts [36]. The hallmark of granulation tissue is the proliferative response of fibroblasts. Proliferation is stimulated by a substance produced by macrophages (growth factor). It is thus very important that the cellular phase (inflammatory phase) is not influenced as to the quality and quantity of the cells. Macrophages are a crucial component of the initial inflammatory reaction which precedes fibroplasia. The administration of corticosteroids in experimental conditions results in significantly fewer monocytes and macrophages in the cellular infiltrate. The effect of fewer macrophages is that the accumulation of collagen – measured as hydroxyproline content – is decreased and neovascularization is inhibited [38].

Fibroblasts proliferate within the first 3 days after trauma. In connection with neovascularization, fibroblasts become the dominating cells in collagen and proteoglycans synthesis. Collagen is also lysed throughout wound repair, perhaps due to fibroblasts. Fibroblasts are responsible for the synthesis of glycosaminglycans, which surrounds the collagen network and absorbs the compressive load as a hydrated viscous gel [27, 30].

Specific Effects of Fibrin, Thrombin, and Factor XIII

Fibrin is vital in wound healing since the network formed in the wound acts both as a scaffold for migrating fibroblasts and as a hemostatic barrier [33]. This scaffold is formed by fibrin strands in connection with fibronectin. In large quantities, fibrin has an inhibitory effect on cell migration and may even delay wound healing. Fibroblasts are quickly followed by new capillaries. These are essential for the granulation tissue. The endothelial cells contain plasminogen activator, the subst-

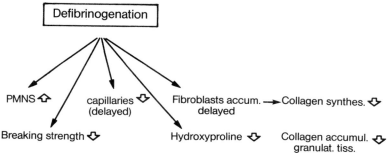

Fig. 5. Effect of defibrinogenation on the different aspects of wound healing

ance that initiates the process of fibrin removal (fibrinolysis). Banerjee and Glynn [5] have demonstrated that implanted fibrin clots are invaded by new capillaries and fibroblasts.

The importance of fibrin in wound repair was confirmed by Brändstedt et al. [7–11]. Defibrinogenation with! Arvin has been used in studies on the formation of granulation tissue (Fig. 5). Under these conditions the fibrin strands are irregular and disrupted, and the number of fibroblasts and collagen fibrils is reduced. As a result of this, a reduction of collagen accumulation in the granulation tissue has been observed. Controlled fibrin deposition appears necessary for granulation tissue formation and for normal healing.

Deposited fibrin apparently stimulates the formation of granulation tissue, including increased collagen precipitation [17]. Hydroxyproline directly reflects the collagen concentration and was significantly high in a fibrin-filled Teflon implanted cylinder [16]. Pohl et al. [34] confirmed the influence of fibrin on growing fibroblasts in vitro by showing that fibrin markedly enhances cellular growth as well as mitosis of the fibroblasts. After 10 days, the cell growth stops. The network of fibrin fibers promotes growth and multiplication of the fibroblasts. As long ago as 1960, Banerjee and Glynn [5] demonstrated that implanted fibrin clots are invaded by new capillaries and fibroblasts.

Thrombin has mitogenic characteristics in cell cultures, aside from its effects on platelet activation, such as long-lasting hormone-like influence on fibroblast proliferation [34], on transformation of factor XIII to XIIIa, on conversion of fibrinogen to fibrin, on prostaglandin production, and on activation of protein C [15]. The effect of thrombin in wound healing is manifold and is a vital part of wound repair.

Factor XIII is needed in the cross-linkage of fibrin in order to produce a stable fibrin network which provides the matrix for the ingrowing fibroblasts. The delay in wound healing in factor XIII-deficient patients may be due to lack of stimulation of fibroblast proliferation [23]. The attachment of fibroblasts is not only obtained by the fibrin matrix, but also (indeed, mainly), through the cross-linkage by activated factor XIII. Cross-linkage between fibrin fibers promotes the cellular response and thus subsequent migration and proliferation of fibroblasts. Factor XIII is also cross-linked with collagen, fibronectin, and α^2-antiplasmin [29].

Fibrin Sealant

For more than 10 years, fibrin sealant (Tissucol/Tisseel), a two-component sealant, has been widely used in surgical medicine and its disciplines.

Tissucol has a triple effect on wound healing. Due to its hemostatic effect, hematoma formation is avoided; consequently the lengthy process of absorption and possible organization of the hematoma does not take place and the rather negative influence of the hematoma on the quality of the granulation tissue is also avoided.

As far as the adhesive effect of Tissucol is concerned, critics have repeatedly pointed out its limited adhesive strength, which will not tolerate major stress exposure. It should, however, be remembered that the objective of using fibrin sealant is not confined to sealing severed tissue segments. Proper adaptation of dissociated surfaces is just as important because it ensures smooth wound healing unhampered by an artificial barrier such as is introduced with synthetic sealants.

The third effect of a fibrin sealant, at least as far as Tissucol/Tisseel is concerned, is on the physiological network structure [35]. This fibrin network is an excellent substrate for the ingrowth of fibroblasts, which will be demonstrated in the study below.

Materials and Methods

To determine the effect of Tissucol on the formation of granulation tissue we developed a spongiosa-based granulation tissue model. The model uses blocks of lyophilized Kieler spongiosa. They were decalcified with hydrochlorous acid and fixed with glutaraldehyde to cross-link the collagen structure. The blocks were then subcutaneously implanted into rats. The cavities of the spongiosa were either filled with a substance that influenced local wound healing, e.g., homologous fibrin sealant, or left empty for controls. The spongiosa blocks were removed at certain time intervals. The granulation tissue was biochemically examined after proteolytic removal from the spongiosa, e.g., to determine the DNA and hydroxyproline content. On the other hand, the granulation tissue was morphometrically evaluated following fixation and prepared for electron microscopy using standard techniques. The space filled by granulation tissue within a given time was precisely determined and the composition of the granulation tissue evaluated. With these methods, we determined the quantity of granulation tissue and the cellular (fibroblasts, capillaries) and biochemical (hydroxyproline, DNA) composition. This model seems very useful since no foreign body reaction was seen, in contrast to the reaction frequently observed after cellular sponge implantation according to Hølund [19].

A total of 72 male Wistar rats were distributed into four equally sized groups. The animals were given intramuscular anesthesia with Ketalar-Rompun, and some of them then received adriamycin (6 mg/kg body weight) before implantation of the spongiosa blocks. All animals underwent paravertebral implantation of two sterile spongiosa blocks with or without fibrin sealant under the dorsal skin. The four groups were thus as follows:

Groups O (F + A): Implantation of spongiosa blocks soaked with fibrin sealant with systemic application of adriamycin.

Group 1 (F): Implantation of spongiosa blocks soaked with fibrin sealant without systemic application of adriamycin.

Group 2 (A): Implantation of spongiosa blocks with systemic application of adriamycin, without fibrin sealant.

Group 3 (CO): Implantation of spongiosa blocks without further systemic or local treatment (control group).

The animals were killed on the 7th or 14th postoperative day.

Results and Discussion

We found a significant fibroblast-stimulating effect of the sealant (16% fibroblasts per volume granulation tissue in controls, 22% in the fibrin sealant group without adriamycin). As opposed to this, the inhibitory effect of the cytostatic agent adriamycin on the formation of granulation tissue was not improved by the sealant (11% without and 10% with sealant). As a cytotoxic chemotherapeutic drug, adriamycin inhibits wound repair. It causes inflammatory arrest, suppresses protein synthesis, and inhibits cell replication [6].

On the electron micrograph, immature (undifferentiated) cells were seen in the adriamycin group (Fig. 6). After 7 days, fibrin strands were markedly visible (Fig. 7), as against the pure fibrin sealant group, in which the fibrin was largely

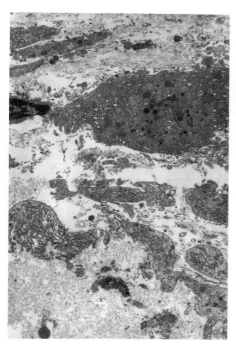
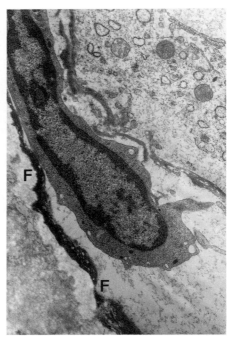

Fig. 6. Immature (undifferentiated) cells in granulation tissue of adriamycin-treated rats (7 days after implantation of spongiosa blocks). EM, x5 000

Fig. 7. Seven days after implantation – fibrin strands (*F*) of applied sealant are still visible in the adriamycin group

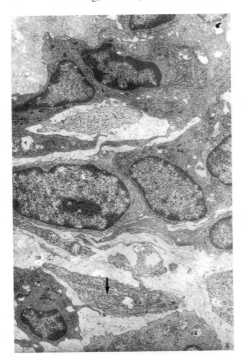

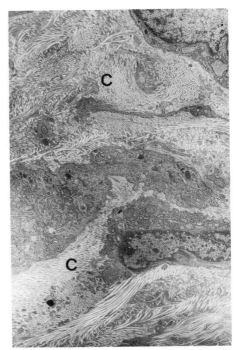

Fig. 8. Without adriamycin application fibrin is completely degraded after 7 days; mature cells are seen in which rough endoplasmic reticulum is already visible (*arrow*)

Fig. 9. Two weeks after implantation a marked collagen (*C*) structure is visible in the Tissucol group, which cannot be observed after adriamycin application

degraded (Fig. 8). After 2 weeks, a marked collagen structure was seen in the fibrin sealant group (Fig. 9); such a structure was not observed in the adriamycin-fibrin sealant group. In the latter group, many collagen-free zones were seen around the fibroblasts, as compared with a dense network of collagen fibers along the fibroblasts in the fibrin sealant group, which also showed abundant granular endoplasmic reticulum, corresponding to type B fibroblasts [1], as described in healing rat and human wounds [37].

It stands to reason that fibrin sealant cannot act on wound healing when cytotoxic drugs are applied simultaneously, since the fibroblasts are directly damaged. Nevertheless, in contrast to these findings, it has been shown that other forms of disturbed wound healing, such as ulcus cruris, can be cured by fibrin sealant in clinical settings, even when the ulcera have been unresponsive to other kinds of treatment [18].

References

1. Aho HJ, Viljanto J, Raekallo J, Pelliniemi LJ (1983) Ultra-structural characteristics of cells in human wound collected by cellstic device. J Surg Res 35: 498–506
2. Baier RE (1972) Surface chemistry in epidermal repair. In: Maibach HI, Rovee DT (eds) Epidermal wound healing. Year Book Medical Publishers, Inc, Chicago, pp. 27–48
3. Balleisen L, Gay S, Marx R, Kühn K (1975) Comparative investigation on the influence of human bovine collagen types I, II and III on the aggregation of human platelets. Klin Wochenschr 53: 903–905
4. Banda MJ, Knighton DR, Hunt TK, Werb Z (1982) Isolation of a nonmitogenic angiogenesis factor from wound fluid. Proc Natl Acad Sci. USA (Cell Biol) 79: 7773–7777
5. Banerjee SK, Glynn LE (1960) Reactions to homologous and heterologous fibrin implants in experimental animals. Ann N Y Acad Sci 86: 1054–1057
6. Bland KI, Palin WE, von Fraunhofer JA, Morris RR, Adcock RA, Tobin GR (1984) Experimental and clinical observations of the effects of cytotoxic chemotherapeutic drugs on wound healing. Ann Surg 199: 782–790
7. Brändstedt S, Olson PS (1980) Effect of defibrinogenation on wound strength and collagen formation. A study in the rabbit. Acta Chir Scand 146: 483–486
8. Brändstedt S, Olson PS (1981) Lack of influence on collagen accumulation in granulation tissue with delayed defibrinogenation. A study in the rabbit. Acta Chir Scand 147: 89–91
9. Brändstedt S, Olson PS, Ahonen J (1980) Effect of defibrinogenation on collagen synthesis in granulation tissue. A study in the rabbit. Acta Chir Scand 146: 551–553
10. Brändstedt S, Rank F, Olson PS (1980) Wound healing and formation of granulation tissue in normal and defibrinogenated rabbits. An experimental model and histological study. Eur surg Res 12: 12–21
11. Brändstedt S, Rank F, Olson PS, Ahonen J (1980) Cell composition of granulation tissue in defibrinogenated rabbits. Acta Chir Scand 146: 545–549
12. Clark RA, Stone RD, Leung DYK, Silver I, Hohn DC, Hunt TK: Role of macrophages in wound healing. Surg Forum 27: 16–18
13. Dhall TZ, Shah GA, Ferguson IA, Dhall DP (1983) Fibrin network structure: modification by platelets. Thromb Haemostas 49: 42–46
14. Greenberg GB, Hunt TK (1978) The proliferative response in vitro of vascular endothelial and smooth muscle cells exposed to wound fluids and macrophages. J Cell Physiol 97: 353–360
15. Gustafson GT (1984) Ecology of wound healing in the oral cavity. Scand J Haematol 33, Suppl. 40: 393–409
16. Hedelin H, Johansson S, Peterson HI, Teger-Nilsson AC, Pettersson S (1982) Influence of fibrin clots on development of granulation tissue in preformed cavities. Surg Gynecol Obstet 154: 521–525
17. Hedelin H, Lundholm K, Teger-Nilsson AC, Peterson HI, Pettersson S (1983) Influence of local fibrin deposition on granulation tissue formation. A biochemical study in the rat. Eur surg Res 15: 312–316 (1983)
18. Holm J (in press) Tisseel skin transplants in leg ulcers. In: Schlag G, Redl H (eds) Fibrin sealant in operative medicine. Plastic, maxillofacial and dental surgery. Springer Berlin Heidelberg New York
19. Hølund B, Junker P, Garbasch C, Christoffersen P, Lorenzen I (1979) Formation of granulation tissue in subcutaneously implanted sponges in rats. Acta path microbiol scand Sect A 87: 367–374
20. Hörmann H, Kühn K (1977) Das Zusammenspiel von humoralen Faktoren, extrazellulärer Matrix und von Zellen bei der Wundheilung. Fortschr Med 95: 1299–1304
21. Hunt TK, Knighton DR, Thakral KK, Goodson WH, Andres WS (1984) Studies on inflammation and wound healing: angiogenesis and collagen synthesis stimulated in vivo by resident and activated wound macrophages. Surgery 86: 48–54
22. Irvin TT (1981) Wound healing. Principles and practice. Chapman and Hall Publ London, New York
23. Kasai S, Kunimoto R, Nitta K (1983) Cross-linking of fibrin by activated factor XIII stimulates attachment, morphological changes and proliferation of fibroblasts. Biomed Res 4: 155–160

24. Key AB, Pepper DS, Ewart MR (1973) Generation of chemotactic activity for leukocytes by the action of thrombin on human fibrinogen. Nature 243: 56–57
25. Knighton DR, Hunt TK, Thakral KK, Goodson WH (1982) Role of platelets and fibrin in the healing sequence. An in vivo study of angiogenesis and collagen synthesis. Ann Surg 196: 379–388
26. Knighton DR, Oredsson S, Banda M, Hunt TK (1984) Regulation of repair: hypoxic control of macrophage mediated angiogenesis. In: Hunt TK, Heppenstall RB, Pines E, Rovee D (eds) Soft and hard tissue repair. Biological and clinical aspects. Praeger Scientific, New York, Philadelphia, Eastbourne 1984, pp 41–49
27. Lehto M, Järvinen M (1985) Collagen and glycosaminoglycan synthesis of injured gastrocnemius muscle in rat. Eur surg Res 17: 179–185
28. Leibovich SJ, Ross R (1976) A macrophage-dependent factor that stimulates the proliferation of fibroblasts in vitro. Am J Pathol 84: 501–513
29. Mishima Y, Nagao F, Ishibiki K, Matsuda M, Nakamura N (1984) Faktor XIII in der Behandlung postoperativer therapie-refraktärer Wundheilungsstörungen. Ergebnisse einer kontrollierten Studie. Chirurg 55: 803–808
30. Minns RJ, Soden PD, Jackson DS (1973) The role of the fibrous components and ground substance in the mechanical properties of biological tissues: a preliminary investigation. J Biochem 6: 153–165
31. Niinikoski J (1969) Effect of oxygen supply on wound healing and formation of experimental granulation tissue. Acta Physiol Scand Suppl 334: 1–72
32. Niinikoski J (1980) Cellular and nutritional interactions in healing wounds. Med Biol 58: 303–309
33. Peacock EE (1984) Inflammation and the cellular response to injury. In: Wound repair, 3rd edn. W.B. Saunders Company, Philadelphia, London, Toronto, pp 1–14
34. Pohl J, Bruhn HD, Christophers E (1979) Thrombin and fibrin-induced growth of fibroblasts: role in wound repair and thrombus organization. Klin Wschr 57: 273–277
35. Redl H, Schlag G, Dinges HP (1985) Vergleich zweier Fibrinkleber. Einfluß ionischer Zusätze auf Fibrinstruktur sowie Morphologie und Wachstum menschlicher Fibroblasten. Med Welt 36: 769–776
36. Ross R (1980) Inflammation, cell proliferation, and connective tissue formation in wound repair. In: Hunt TK (ed) Wound healing and wound infection. Theory and surgical practice. Appleton Century Crofts, New York, p 1–8
37. Ross R, Odland G (1968) Human wound repair. II. Inflammatory cells, epithelia–mesenchymal interrelations, and fibrogenesis. J Cell Biol 39: 152–164
38. Salmela K, Roberts PJ, Lautenschlager I, Ahonen J (1980) The effect of local methylprednisolone on granulation tissue formation. II. Mechanisms of action. Acta Chir Scand 146: 541–544

Fibrin Sealant and Its Modes of Application

H. REDL, and G. SCHLAG

Key words: antibiotics, collagen fleece, Duploject system, fibrin glue, hemostasis, spray, tissue adhesive, tissue sealing, wound healing

Abstract

After reconstitution, the two components of fibrin sealant – sealer protein/aprotinin and thrombin/CaCl$_2$ solution – can be applied in different ways. Besides sequential application or premixing of the reactant, application of the sealant components with the double-syringe applicator (Duploject) is advantageous in a number of ways, e.g., single-handed operation, thorough mixing, thin-layer application. Use of the Duploject is almost universally applicable. Thrombin concentration can be varied depending on the need for rapid or slow clotting of the sealants. The sealant can be delivered using needles, spray heads, or catheters, as indicated by the specific application. The spraying catheter can be easily used through the biopsy channel of an endoscope. Furthermore special micro-application techniques are possible. Fibrin sealant may also be used in connection with other biomaterials such as collagen (fleece), dura, and vascular grafts. Tests are reported on different collagen fleeces as well as on the addition of antibiotics. Finally visibility (including X-ray) and histological techniques are discussed.

The Material

Fibrin sealant is available under the trade names Tissucol, Tisseel, or Fibrin-kleber Human Immuno as a kit containing freeze-dried powder, freeze-dried thrombin, calcium chloride, and aprotinin solution. The substances mix to form two components: sealer and thrombin solution. To prepare the sealer, protein concentrate is dissolved in the accompanying stock solution of fibrinolysis inhibitor (aprotinin 3000 KIU/ml) or a dilution of it, where applicable. To simplify and speed up reconstitution (5–10) min of the highly concentrated sealer proteins, we developed a combined heating and stirring device – Fibrinotherm (Fig. 1). Thrombin is reconstituted in the accompanying 40 mM of calcium chloride solution, to yield concentrations of either 500 or 4 (NIH) units (NIH-U) of thrombin per milliliter depending on the chosen method of application. As the two components combine during application, fibrin sealant consolidates and adheres to the site of application, i.e., to the tissue.

The most important of the sealer proteins is fibrinogen, whose molecular weight is about 340 000 daltons. The molecule consists of six polypeptide chains of three different types – α, β, and γ. Through the action of thrombin, the fibrinopeptides A

Fibrin Sealant in Operative Medicine
Traumatology and Orthopaedics – Vol. 7
Edited by G. Schlag, H. Redl
© Springer-Verlag Berlin Heidelberg 1986

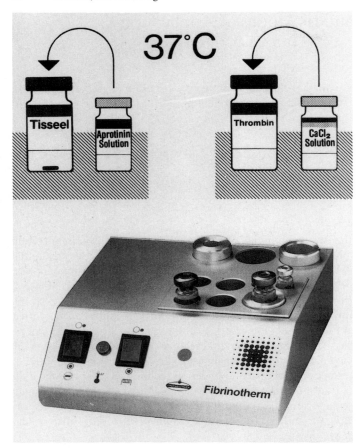

Fig. 1. Component preparation – Fibrinotherm

and B are split off from the resulting fibrin monomer. These fibrin monomers aggregate largely because of hydrogen bonding and thus produce the resulting fibrin clot. These reactions duplicate the last phase of the clotting cascade (Fig. 2). The time required for the onset of coagulation is dependent on the amount of thrombin used.

To achieve maximal tensile strength, cross-linking between fibrin α-chains is necessary. Fibrin seal itself contains sufficient factor XIII (which is activated by thrombin) to produce a high degree of cross-linking; the latter proceeds slowly, but the initial steepness of the α-cross-linkage curve results in sufficient tensile strength after about 3–5 min. In previous studies [1, 2], we were able to demonstrate the direct dependency of tensile strength on α-chain cross-linking. In other experiments [3, 4] we found that the intrinsic tensile strength of a clot formed with fibrin seal was about 1200 g/cm^2 (157 kPa) while that of a sealed rat skin was approximately 200 g/cm^2 (17 kPa) after 10 min cross-linking at 37°C, implying that adhesion of the sealant

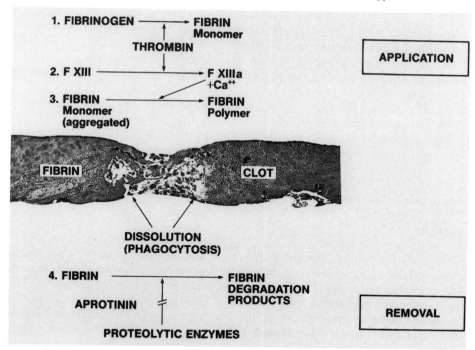

Fig. 2. Fibrin clot formation and removal

to the tissue is the decisive factor for gluing tissue. The adhesive qualities of consolidated fibrin sealant to the tissue might be explainable in terms of covalent bonding between fibrin and collagen [5] or fibrin, fibronectin, and collagen.

As far as the adhesive effect is concerned, critics have repeatedly pointed out its limited adhesive strength compared with synthetic acrylate adhesives. This is compensated for by the high elasticity of the material [6], which makes the material especially useful for nonstatic tissue, e.g., lung parenchyma. In addition, applications onto wet surfaces are equally possible, as is shown in Table 1. However, the applications of fibrin sealant are not limited to sealing severed tissue segments, as adequate hemostasis is also achieved.

Table 1. Tensile strength of sealed rabbit skin in relation to tissue moisture before application of Tisseel (method similar to that described by Redl et al.[26]

Dry (with pads)	Wet (with Ringer's solution)
× 48.2 g STD ± 10.7	53.3 g ± 12.8

To a variable extent, sealant persistence in vivo can be controlled by adding an antifibrinolytic agent [7]. Previous studies have demonstrated that aprotinin, a natural antiprotease, is superior to synthetic antifibrinolytic agents [8]; this has been confirmed by other reports [9]. Sealant degradation rate depends on

a) the fibrinolytic (or more generally the proteolytic) activity in the area of application,
b) the thickness of the sealant layer – which should be as thin as possible – and
c) the amount of aprotinin present.

Thus expected clot persistence can only be dealt with on an individualized basis. However, excessively long survival of the sealant may not be desirable [10].

Application of Fibrin Sealant

General

Historically the components were applied sequentially with relatively poor mixing owing to fast buildup of fibrin membranes between them. This prompted us to study mixing ratios, and alternative application techniques and their effects on the seal produced. Ever since the first applications of fibrin sealant the strength obtainable has been known to depend both on the fibrinogen concentration [11] and on the amount of cross-linkage [8]. Using a design for measuring intrinsic clot strength [3], we tried to find the optimum mixing ratio [12]. The mixture of one part sealant and one part thrombin solution gave the best results, although thorough mixing appears to be the decisive factor.

The gross and microscopic data obtained from experiments on rat skin revealed [12] that seals produced with premixed reactants (4 NIH-U thrombin/ml) or with the Duploject applicator (4 or 500 NIH-U/ml) had a superior tensile strength to those obtained with sequential application of reactants. There is no doubt that cavitation, as observed microscopically, is one factor involved. Another factor is insufficient availability of the reactants at the reaction site, since adequate cross-linkage requires a minimum concentration of Ca^{2+} [13], which may not be achieved locally if mixing is incomplete.

Duploject System with Needle

While we have repeatedly stressed the disadvantages associated with sequential application (poor mixing and cumbersome handling) [8, 12], the technique has not lost its role in selected cases, e.g., in combination with collagen fleece or vascular graft material so as to facilitate mixing.

In most cases, application of the sealant components with the double-syringe applicator (Duploject) is advantageous, e.g., single-handed operation, thorough mixing, and thin-layer applications. Use of the Duploject is almost universally applicable (Fig. 3).

Low thrombin concentrations (4 NIH-U/ml – slow clotting) are beneficial in all those applications where the parts to be sealed require subsequent adaptation, e.g.,

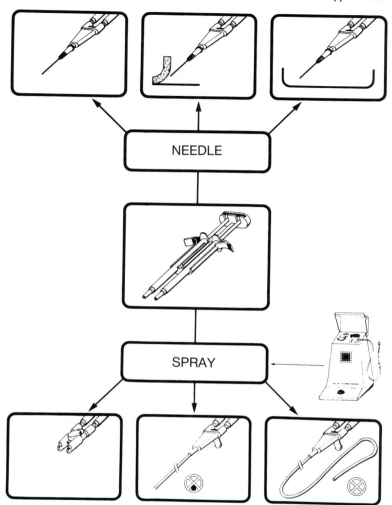

Fig. 3. Duploject system

in skin grafting and in some microsurgical operations. If, however, hemostasis is of primary interest, a high thrombin concentration, i.e., 500 NIH-U/ml, should be used as this ensures almost instantaneous clotting.

The double-syringe unit with mixing attachment – needle or catheter – is designed for simultaneous operation of the two barrels so that the two components are ejected at the same time but separately via the exchangeable mixing needle. As long as the sealant is being applied, there will be no clogging of the needle. Once application is interrupted, insertion of a new needle makes the applicator ready for use again.

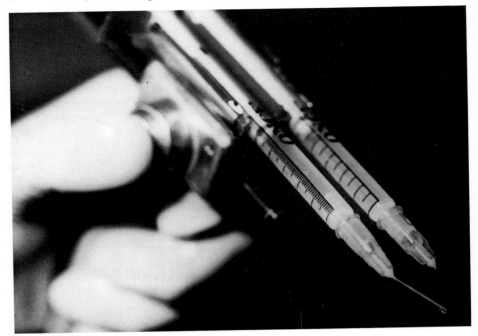

a

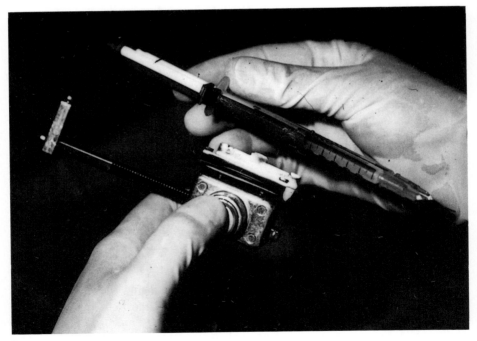

b

Fig. 4 a, b. Microapplicator to be used with Duploject system

Certain operations require the use of a microapplicator (Fig. 4) which allows repeated application of the same small volume per ejection; this is especially useful when using 4 NIH-U thrombin per milliliter. A similar system was developed by Tange [14]. An alternative is to mix the two components on a piece of aluminum foil and apply the premixed sealant with a spatula [15]. To get an "ultramicro" dosing (but without mixing) the special device of Chüden [16] may be used.

Duploject System – Spray Applications

The spray head or spray catheter (lower part of Fig. 3) is connected to a conventional pressurized gas source. The gas pressure is reduced to 2 bar (head) or 4 bar (catheter) in order to obtain a gas flow of 5–10 liters/min, which is optimum for use with the Tissomat (Fig. 3). The two components are injected separately into the continuous gas jet. The optimal distance between the spray head and the wound surface is approximately 10 cm for the head and 1 cm for the catheter. As the droplets bombard each other in the air and on the wound surface, they mix, and at a high thrombin concentration instantly form a delicate fibrin film. A thin film so produced is optimum and is required for the sealant to promote wound healing [10]. Spray head application also allows coating of extensive surfaces with a small amount of sealant. Thus an area of about 100 cm^2 can be coated with the 1-ml kit.

The spray head is especially useful for covering large areas, e.g., resected surfaces of parenchymal organs [17], for fixation of skin grafts and coating the donor area [18, 19], and for hemostasis of diffuse epicardial bleeding [20].

In the four-lumen spray catheter (Fig. 5), two lumens are used for the components, the third one for the gas, and in the short version a malleable wire is contained within the fourth lumen. The "spray catheter" can also be used, without spraying gas, to mix the two components in an otherwise inaccessible area, e.g., an esophageal-bronchopleural fistula [21]. In the latter case, the third lumen may be used to apply X-ray contrast dye for catheter localization.

Catheter spray systems can be modified to seal otherwise inaccessible areas by either:

1. The use of endoscopy (with biopsy channels) and a 150-cm-catheter (Figs. 5, 7), or
2. The short catheter with a malleable wire which allows any specific catheter shape (Fig. 6).

These catheters may be used for pleurodesis in recurrent pneumothorax [22–24], to occlude bronchopleural [25], rectovaginal, and esophageal-bronchopleural fistulas [26], to arrest gastric [27] and esophageal bleeding to ensure tissue sealing of the larynx, to fix flaps in plastic surgery, and to achieve hemostasis in epistaxis and after prostatectomy. An additional advantage offered by spraying with the Duploject spray is that the gas jet can be operated separately and can be used to clean and dry the operating site. The sealant is thus applied to a "dry" surface, which facilitates hemostasis. In addition, no clogging occurs when the sealing procedure is interrupted.

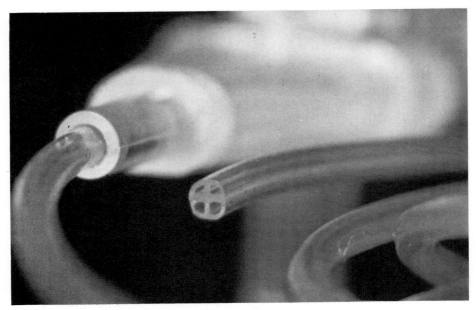

Fig. 5. Spray catheter with characteristic four-lumen design

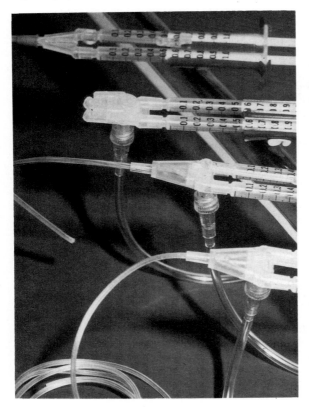

Fig. 6. Spray adaptors of the Duploject system

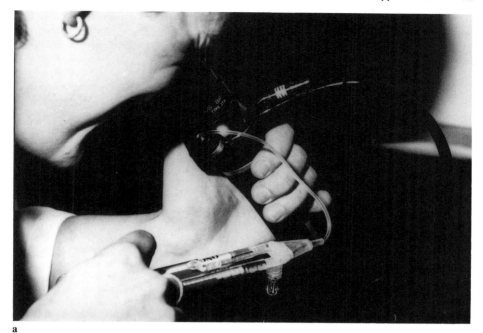

a

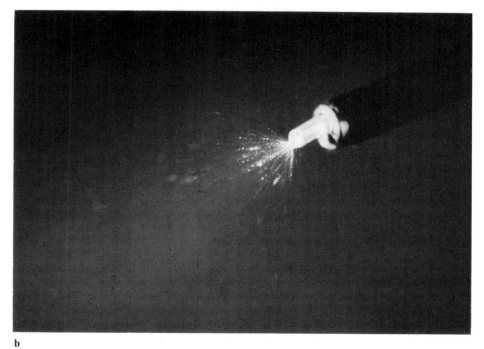

b

Fig. 7a u. b. Use of spray catheter through the biopsy channel of the endoscope. **a** Insertion into the channel. **b** Catheter in action, fibrin coming out of the biopsy channel at the tip of the bronchoscope

A cut Swan-Ganz catheter can also be used, as outlined by Linscheer [28]. This technique [15] has been successfully employed to treat patients with pneumothorax [29].

Combination of Fibrin Sealant with Matrices

For some applications the additional use of sealant support, e.g., Dacron patches, lyophilized dura, fascia, or collagen fleece, proved useful. However, not all of the commercially available fleeces are suitable for this purpose, and preliminary tests are therefore mandatory before clinical use. Some fleeces were tested by Stemberger [9] to assess their effects on platelet aggregation. We feel that pliable collagen fleeces are best suited for this purpose. Therefore we performed a preliminary study with some of the available fleeces. Test criteria were:

1. Uptake of liquid
2. Tensile strength in the wet state
3. Ease in handling
4. Tissue reactivity

Preliminary Results

1. To test the absorption of water, 1×1 cm pieces of collagen fleece of different thickness were used (for results, see Table 2). Absorption of H_2O was negligible with Collatamp and slow with Gelfix, all other fleeces absorbed H_2O immediately, which seems to be of essential importance in ensuring adequate soaking with sealant components. Some of the fleeces absorbed H_2O differently at the upper and the lower surfaces.
2. There were great differences in tensile strength in wet conditions (Table 2). Gelfix showed the highest tensile strength of all the fleeces tested. As expected, the Braun fleece had negligible tensile strength, whereas the Helitrex fleece of only 3 mm showed a remarkable tensile strength of 40–50 g.
3. Most of the collagen fleeces were easy to work with in wet conditions, with the exception of the Braun fleece, which broke into pieces and stuck to the gloves. (However, after our examinations had been completed, an improved fleece was developed.) The application of collagen fleece in dry conditions deserves special

Table 2. Test criteria and results of tests on different collagen fleeces in vitro

Company	Hydrophilic surface	Tensile strength	Handling	Tissue reaction
Braun	+	2 g	−	∅
Collatamp	−	10 g	+/−	+
Gelfix	−	150 g	−	+
Pentapharm	+	15 g	+/−	+/−
Helitrex	+	55 g	+	+/−
Savolon	+	50 g (inhomogeneous)	+	∅

mention, especially in regard to spray applications. The only fleeces suitable for this mode of application are Helitrex and Savolon 3 mm, whose properties with regard to ease of handling and H$_2$O absorption (in particular rapidity and volume of absorption of water) are excellent.

4. For histological examination, moistened pieces of fleece (size: 1×0.5 mm) were applied subcutaneously in rats according to a similar model of wound healing used by Rudas [30]. Blinding evaluation was performed after 14 days. The findings may be summarized as follows: In principle, every fleece tested was still detectable after 14 days; the larger pieces, however, were less disintegrated. The loosely textured Braun fleece and Savolon were absorbed relatively rapidly. The foreign body reaction seemed relatively limited with Braun, Savolon, Pentapharm and Helitrex, while Gelfix and Collatamp cause a more severe reaction. In view of our experience thus far, we recommend the use of Helitrex as a standard fleece for fibrin sealing. In addition to its properties outlined above, it has a further special property: if pressed in a dry condition it may be greatly compressed, yet when absorbing liquid, e.g., fibrin sealant, it expands to its original dimensions. This may result in interesting applications, e.g., endoscopy.

Combination of fibrin sealant with either decalcified bone (ongoing studies in this laboratory) or hydroxyapatite (see orthopedic section) is a further example of heterogenic combination. Fibrin sealant may also be used to fix bioprostheses, such as the middle ear bones [31].

Combination of Fibrin Seal with Antibiotics

The practice has been to apply fibrin seal only to areas unlikely to become infected. To overcome this limitation, the addition of antibiotics to the fibrin seal seemed desirable. As early as 1950 a patent was described in the USA in which the combined application of fibrin and antibiotics was used [32]. Fibrin seal has also been used in combination with antibiotics both experimentally and clinically [33, 34]. Therefore we studied the in vitro properties of mixtures of fibrin seal and antibiotics, particularly their effect on coagulation time, cross-linking, and drug release [3, 4].

For the practical application of fibrin seal, it is important to note that the clotting time can be regulated by the use of higher thrombin concentrations and the rate of fibrin-α-chain cross-linkage with additional factor XIII. Drug release from fibrin seal is probably by simple diffusion, and therefore to a large extent, dependent on the concentration gradient between the clot and its environment. This implies that although antibiotics incorporated into fibrin clots are retained for longer than when they are directly instilled into body cavities, drug retention is much lower than with bone cement-antibiotic mixtures and is insufficient to maintain adequate local drug concentrations for more than 3 days. This observation has also been confirmed in a recent in vivo study [35]. The limitations may be overcome by newer, less soluble antibiotics [36]. Nevertheless, infections may be controlled in the early stages after bone surgery using fibrin seal containing relatively high antibiotic concentrations. However, the total dose of drug should be less than the recommended maximal daily systemic dose.

Detection of Fibrin Seal in Tissues

Owing to the opaque white appearance of coagulated fibrin sealant, it is usually easy to detect fibrin in the sealing area. However, for special indications (e.g., in eye surgery) or with sequential application, in which one might wish to observe the delivery of the sealer protein solution, adding disulphine blue dye (ICI) (10 µl/ml sealer protein solution) is effective in rendering the fibrin seal visible.

For X-ray detection the addition of different contrast media was tested by Richling [37]. Metrizamide was found to be superior, but its general use cannot be recommended because of slight depression of fibrin-α-chain cross-linking.

Reviews on histological techniques for identifying fibrin sealant have been published by Dinges [30] and Heine [38]. With the phosphotungstic acid method of Mallory and the trichrome technique of Lendrum it is possible to visualize easily the fibrin sealant with light microscopy, but the fibrin sealant does not react as well as endogenous fibrin (perhaps due to the thicker network of fibrin strands). The histological differentiation between exogenous fibrin sealant and endogenous fibrin requires some experience if standard fibrin techniques are employed. If heterologous fibrin glue is used in animal experiments, its demonstration with the immunoperoxidase technique gives optimal results [30]. It is also easily seen with hematoxylin-eosin stain and shows up nicely on trichrome stain.

Conclusions

In summary, for the optimal use of fibrin sealant the application technique should meet the following requirements [12].
1. The sealant components should be fully dissolved and kept at a temperature of 37°C (which is easy with the Fibrino thermsystem — Fig. 7).
2. The wound surfaces should be as dry as possible (though application to wet surfaces is feasible).
3. The components should be thoroughly mixed on application.
4. The thrombin and aprotinin concentrations may be adjusted to the purpose of application.
5. The sealant should be applied as a thin film.
6. After clotting has occurred, further mechanical stresses should be avoided for about 3–5 min because of the time course of α-chain cross-linking.

Fibrin sealant is useful in controlling microvascular or capillary bleeding from ruptured or surgically dissected tissues. It is particularly beneficial in patients with increased bleeding tendencies undergoing surgery. It might also be used to seal tissue with different kinds of biomaterials. Thus fibrin sealant has a place in all surgical disciplines for the purposes of tissue sealing, hemostasis, and support of wound healing. There seem to be few drawbacks, not even such as the risk of viral transmittance [39, 40]; however, the benefits of combining fibrin sealing with modern-day surgery far outweigh any known risks.

References

1. Guttmann J (1979) Untersuchung eines Fibrinklebers für die Anwendung in der Chirurgie peripherer Nerven. Diplomarbeit, Technische Universität Wien
2. Seelich T, Redl H (1980) Theoretische Grundlagen des Fibrinklebers. In: Schimpf K (ed) Fibrinogen, Fibrin und Fibrinkleber. FK Schattauer-Verlag, Stuttgart, New York (1980) 199–208
3. Redl H, Stanek G, Hirschl A, Schlag G (1982), Fibrinkleber-Antibiotika-Gemische – Festigkeit und Elutionsverhalten. In: Cotta H, Braun A (eds) Fibrinkleber in Orthopädie und Traumatologie. Georg Thieme Verlag, Stuttgart, New York, pp 18–21
4. Redl H, Schlag G, Stanek G, Hirschl A, Seelich T (1983) In vitro properties of mixtures of fibrin seal and antibiotics. Biomaterials 4: 29–32
5. Duckert F, Nyman D, Gastpar H (1978) Factor XIII fibrin and collagen. Coll Platelet Interact., FK Schattauer-Verlag, Stuttgart, New York, pp 391–396
6. Redl H, Schlag G (1986) Properties of different tissue sealants with special emphasis on fibrinogen based preparations. In: Schlag G, Redl H (eds) Fibrin sealant in Operative Medicine. Springer-Verlag, Heidelberg, Berlin, this volume
7. Pflüger H, Redl H (1982) Abbau von Fibrinkleber in vivo und in vitro (Versuche an der Ratte mit besonderer Berücksichtigung der klinischen Relevanz). Z Urol Nephrol 75: 25–30
8. Redl H, Schlag G, Dinges HP, Kuderna H, Seelich T (1982) Background and methods of fibrin sealing. In: Winter D, Gibbons DF, Plenk H (eds) Biomaterials. John Wiley and Sons Ltd (1982) 669–676
9. Stemberger A, Fritsche HM, Haas S, Spilker G, Wriedt-Lübbe I, Blümel G (1982) Biochemische und experimentelle Aspekte der Gewebeversiegelung mit Fibrinogen und Kollagen. In: Cotta H, Braun A (eds) Fibrinkleber in Orthopädie und Traumatologie. Georg Thieme Verlag, Stuttgart, New York, pp 290–293
10. Schlag G, Redl H, Thurnher M, Dinges HP (1986) The importance of fibrin in wound repair. In: Schlag G, Redl H (eds) Principles of fibrin sealant. Springer-Verlag, Heidelberg, Berlin, in press
11. Matras H, Dinges HP, Lassmann H, Mamoli B (1972) Zur nahtlosen interfaszikulären Nerventransplantation im Tierexperiment. Wr Med Wschr 122: 517
12. Redl H, Schlag G, Dinges HP (1982) Methods of fibrin seal application. Thorac Cardiovasc Surg 30: 223–227
13. Seelich T, Redl H (1979) Biochemische Grundlagen zur Klebemethode. Dtsch Z Mund-Kiefer-Gesichtschir 3: 22S–26S
14. Tange RA (1986) A new application method for fibrin sealant: glue gun. In: Schlag G, Redl H (eds) Fibrin sealant in Operative Medicine – otorhinolaryngology. Springer-Verlag, Heidelberg, Berlin, this volume
15. Redl H, Schlag G (1984) Background and methods of fibrin sealing. In: Skjoldborg H (ed) Scientific Workshop '82: Tisseel/Tissucol-Symposium – Areas of application, problems and perspectives in current surgery. Immuno Denmark, pp 11–19
16. Chüden HG (1986) Simplified application of fibrinous glue in middle-ear surgery. In: Schlag G, Redl H (eds) Fibrin sealant in Operative Medicine – otorhinolaryngology. Springer-Verlag Heidelberg, Berlin, this volume
17. Servadio L (1983) Tisseal in liver surgery. (Film)
18. Pers M (1984) Scand. J. Plast. Reconstr. Surg. 17: 178
19. Riedmiller H, Thüroff JW (1985). In: Melchior H (ed.) Fibrinklebung in der Urologie. Springer-Verlag, Berlin Heidelberg New York, pp 71–76
20. Haverich A, Walterbusch G, Oelert H, Borst HG (1984) In: Scheele J (ed.) Fibrinklebung, Springer-Verlag, Berlin Heidelberg New York, pp 143–149
21. Pridun N, Heindl W, Redl H, Schlag G, Machacek E (1986) In: Schlag G, Redl H (eds) Fibrin sealant in operative medicine, Springer-Verlag, Heidelberg, this volume
22. Jessen C, Sharma P (1985) Ann. Thorac. Surg. 39: 521
23. Pridun N, Heindl W (1983) Wr. Klin. Wochenschr. 133, Suppl. 75: 40
24. Buchwald J (1984) In: Scheele J (ed.) Fibrinklebung, Springer-Verlag, Heidelberg Berlin, New York, pp 169–172

25. Waclawiczek H, Wayand W, Chmelicek A (1986) In: Schlag G, Redl H (eds.) Fibrin sealant in operative medicine, Springer-Verlag, Heidelberg, this volume
26. Flicker M, Pesendorf FX, Redl H (1985) Wr. Med. Wochenschrift 135, Suppl. 90:21
27. Armengol JR (1985) In: Schlag G, Redl H (eds.) Fibrin sealant in operative medicine, Springer-Verlag, Heidelberg, this volume
28. Linscheer WG, Fazio TL (1979) Control of upper gastrointestinal hemorrhage by endoscopic spraying of clotting factor. Gastroenterology 77: 642–645
29. Pridun N, Heindl W (1983) Fibrinspraytherapie beim Spontanpneumothorax. Wr Klin Wochenschr 133, Suppl 75: 40
30. Dinges HP, Redl H, Schlag G (1982) Histologische Techniken und tierexperimentelle Modelle zur Untersuchung der Wechselwirkung zwischen Fibrinkleber und Gewebe. In: Cotta H, Braun A (eds) Fibrinkleber in Orthopädie und Traumatologie. Georg Thieme Verlag, Stuttgart, New York, pp 44–51
31. Siedentop KH, Harris D, Loewy A (1983) Experimental use of fibrin tissue adhesive in middle ear surgery. Laryngoscope 93: 1 310–1 313
32. Ferry JD, Morrison PR (1950) Fibrin clots and methods for preparing the same. United States Patent, Dec 5, 2,533,004
33. Braun A, Schumacher G, Kratzat R, Heine WD, Pasch B (1980) Der Fibrin-Antibiotika-Verband im Tierexperiment zur lokalen Therapie des Staphylokokken infizierten Knochens. H Unfallheilkunde 148: 809
34. Bösch P, Lintner F, Braun F (1979) Die autologe Spongiosatransplantation unter Anwendung des Fibrinklebesystems im Tierexperiment. Wr Klin Wochenschr 91: 628
35. Stanek G, Bösch P, Weber P, Hirschl A (1980) Experimentelle Untersuchungen für das pharmakokinetische Verhalten lokal applizierter Antibiotika. Acta Med Austriaca 4, Suppl 20: 19
36. Wahlig H, Dingeldein E, Braun A, Kratzat R (1982) Fibrinkleber und Antibiotika – Untersuchungen zur Freisetzungskinetik. In: Cotta H, Braun A (eds) Fibrinkleber in Orthopädie und Traumatologie, Georg Thieme Verlag, Stuttgart, New York, pp 182
37. Richling B (1982) Homologous controlled-viscosity fibrin for endovascular embolization. Part. I: Experimental development of the medium. Acta Neurochir 62: 159
38. Heine WD, Braun A, Edinger D (1982) Gewebliche Abwehrreaktionen auf das Fibrinklebesystem. In: Cotta H, Braun A (eds) Fibrinkleber in Orthopädie und Traumatologie. Georg Thieme Verlag, Stuttgart, New York, pp 277
39. Barrett PN, Dorner F, Eibl J (1986) In: Schlag G, Redl H (eds) Fibrin sealant in Operative Medicine. Springer-Verlag, Heidelberg, Berlin, this volume
40. Eder G, Neumann M, Cerwenka R, Baumgarten K. In: Schlag G, Redl H (eds) Fibrin sealant in Operative Medicine. Springer-Verlag, Heidelberg, Berlin, this volume

Properties of Different Tissue Sealants with Special Emphasis on Fibrinogen-Based Preparations

H. Redl, and G. Schlag

Key words: fine clot, coarse clot, fibrin sealant, fibroblast proliferation, tissue adhesive, fibrinogen, wound healing, hemostasis

Abstract

Different tissue sealants are described with special emphasis on the performance of different fibrinogen-based sealants. Therefore the biochemical properties of four different fibrinogen-based tissue adhesives are compared in detail. The major difference is in clot structure – coarse versus fine. Related to this structural difference are additional dissimilar properties. The coarse type fibrin sealant proved to be superior in tensile strength, cell compatibility and fibroblastic proliferation.

Introduction

The use of tissue adhesives as an alternative method for repairing injured tissues, and more importantly, as a means for improving wound healing, may be based either on natural or synthetic materials. Therefore, it is necessary to compare various natural adhesives (e.g. fibrin sealant) to each other, as well as to synthetic preparations (e.g. cyanoacrylates), in order to asses their relative advantages and disadvantages in regards to clinical applicability (Table 1).

Table 1. Tissue Sealants

Synthetic	Natural
Acrylates	(Plasma)
Gelatine-Formaldehyde-Resorcin	(Cryoprecipitate)
	Fibrin Sealant

One obvious advantage of fibrinogen-based materials is their complete degradation and rapid removal from the body. Thus, local and systemic toxicity are avoided.

In the present study, we compare the biochemical properties of four different fibrinogen-based tissue adhesives; in addition, the similarities and differences of these natural adhesives, as compared to synthetic preparations, are discussed (Tables 2, 3).

Fibrin Sealant in Operative Medicine
Traumatology and Orthopaedics – Vol. 7
Edited by G. Schlag, H. Redl
© Springer-Verlag Berlin Heidelberg 1986

Table 2. Advantages and Disadvantages of Fibrin Sealant Versus Acrylates

	Fibrin sealant	Acrylates
Application to wet area	Possible	Impossible
Adhesivity	Good	Better
Elasticity	Very good	None
Tissue compatibility	Excellent	Poor
Absorption or degradation	Complete	None
Hemostasis	Excellent	None
Supporting of wound healing	Obtainable	Unobtainable
Application in bone and cartilage	Possible	Impossible
Foreign granulation tissue	None	Invariably present
Risk of virus infection	None*	None

*according to current knowledge

Table 3. Clottable Material [mg/ml]

Cryoprecipitate	AF	Fibrin sealant
29	11	80

Special emphasis is put on two fibrin sealants, which differ mainly in their ionic composition. Ferry and Morrison [1] described the influence of ionic strength on clot structure in 1947. High ionic strength results in "fine" clots and physiological ionic strength in "coarse" clots.

Material and Methods

The four fibrinogen-based, natural adhesives utilized in the study were cryoprecipitate, autologous fibrin (AF)[2] and two fibrin sealants. One fibrin sealant contains a physiological salt concentration (PS) while the second has a high salt concentration (HS) to achieve fast reconstitution.

Protein concentration and composition, kinetics of fibrin alpha-chain crosslinking, factor XIII content, conductivity and osmolarity were measured as described in Redl et al [3]. Intrinsic strength of the formed fibrin clots was tested in an apparatus similar to the one described by Redl et al]4], but using a 0.2 ml butterfly shaped mould for the breaking strength test and a larger one, 0.8 ml with 1.5 cm usable length, for elasticity measurements. The velocity used for stretching the fibrin clots was 1 cm/min.

Human diploid embryonal lung fibroblasts MRC5 were cultivated and their viability tested as described by Redl et al ([3]. Fibroblast proliferation was evaluated according to Mosmann [5] either on cell layers or in cell suspension using the substrate (3-(4,5 Dimethylthiazol-2-yl)-2,5-Diphenyl Tetrazolium Bromide) (Sigma, USA) (= MTT). The effect of the two fibrin sealants on fibroblasts was assessed in either a liquid or solidified state.

In order to assess the influence, if any, of the liquid sealants on the cells, the latter were seeded into the wells of TC Cluster 24 plates (Coster) and incubated at 37°C under 95% air + 5% CO_2 until an almost uniformly dense cell layer had formed. Following dilution of the sealants with equal volumes of isotonic NaCl solution, the cell cultures were covered with 0.5 ml of sealant solution for a maximum of 30 minutes. The effects of dilute sealants on the cells were observed using light microscopy and the supernatants removed at fixed intervals. The cells were then washed with isotonic NaCl solution and stained with Ziel-Neelsen Carbol Fuchsin (diluted 1:10 with water); micrographs were produced using a Polyvar microscope (Reichert).

The proliferation rate was determined according to Mosmann [5] and was used to obtain quantitative data. After incubation with liquid sealant as described above, 50 μl of MTT (5 mg/ml) was added and incubated further for 2^h at 37°C. Simultaneously 0.1 ml MRC5 cell suspension (5×10^5/ml) was added to 0.1 ml of each sealant solution, incubated for 30 min. and then incubated further at 37°C after the addition of 20μl MTT solution. The reaction was stopped with 0.4 N HCl in 2-propanol and the accumulated dye extracted. Photometric measurements were done after centrifugation of the supernatant fluid (diluted threefold with 0.4 N HCl/2-propanol) at 570 nm. This test has been shown to correlate well with the ^{3}H-thymidin uptake test [5].

In order to assess whether the solidified sealants differed in their influence on fibroblasts and to evaluate the fibrin structure, equal volumes of sealant solution were rapidly mixed at 37°C with thrombin-$CaCl_2$ solution (4 IU of thrombin/ml, 40 mmol of $CaCl_2$/l) and 0.5 ml of the mixture was poured into each TC Cluster 24 plate well (Costar) and incubated at 37°C and 100% rel. humidity for 1 hour. Plasma clots were produced similarly by mixing 0.9 ml of citrated human plasma with 0.1 ml of thrombin-$CaCl_2$ solution (4 IU thrombin/ml, 0.3 mol $CaCl_2$/l).

Some of the sealant clots were washed 4 times, each time with 0.2 ml of isotonic NaCl solution for 20 min at 37°C under continuous agitation; the washing efficiency was checked by washing clots of the same type with distilled water and determining the supernatant conductivity after each washing. The nonwashed clots and those washed with isotonic NaCl solution were each cut at a small angle (to obtain a rougher surface), covered with 0.2 ml MRC5 fibroblast suspension (5×10^5 cells/ml medium), and incubated for 24 hours at 37°C under 95% air + 5% CO_2. Direct examination of cells under the light microscope was possible only with the transparent HS fine clots, not with the milky white PS coarse clots. Therefore, the samples were prepared for histologic examination by fixing them in 3.5% formaldehyde solution followed by standard procedures of dehydration and paraffin embedding. For SEM examination, the samples were fixed with 1% glutaraldehyde (cacodylate buffer), refixed with 1% OsO_4, alcohol dehydrated, and critical point dried with CO_2. Dried samples were fractured in order to observe both surface and inner structures and gold sputtered (10 nm, Polaron Sputter) for scanning by a (Jeol-SM 35) SEM at 25 kV accelerating voltage.

Results

Cryoprecipitate and autologuos fibrin (AF) were found to have a low fibrinogen (clottable protein) concentration (Table 3), only moderate α-chain crosslinking (Table 4) and therefore only limited tensile strength (Table 5).

Both fibrin sealants require approximately the same reconstitution time (5–10 min) when PS dissolved at 37°C by using the combined warming and stirring unit described before [3] and HS at room temperature under manual shaking. Dissolution of HS at 37°C reduces the time required to 3–6 min.

PS and HS were found to be identical in their kinetics of fibrin crosslinking (Table 4) if FXIII is added to the latter.

Table 4. Crosslinking of Fibrin α-Chain (% of α-Polymer)

Incubation time (min)	Cryoprecipitate	AF	PS (coarse)	HS (fine)
120	35	36	80	80*

*(with additional factor XIII; see Table 6)

Intrinsic tensile strength was 4 to 5 times higher ($p < 0.001$, Student-t-test) in the PS coarse clots (Table 5). Due to the brittle nature of the HS fine clot, more than 50 % of the specimens broke during manipulation and were therefore excluded from the measurements. For the same reason, we were unable to obtain stress-strain results (length-tension relationships) of fine clots (Fig. 1). The decreased elasticity of the fine clots appeared to be unrelated to the fibrin sealant, as standard fibrin fine clots (with minimal lateral aggregation of protofibrils) were also irreversibly deformed, as compared to coarse type clots [6].

As was the case with fibrin structures, the different effects of solidified sealants on fibroblasts were best visualized on the cut surfaces of clots. On smooth PS clot

Table 5. Intrinsic Strength [g/cm^2] (kPa) (incubation temperature = 37°C)

Incubation time (min)	Cryo	AF	PS	HS
10	198 45* (19kPa) n=7	237 (23kPa) n=2	616+101 (60kPa) n=5	
30		not investigated	899+155* (88kPa) n=8	192+41** (19kPa) n=8

 * = signif. p. < 0.001 Student t-Test
** = 50% of the fine clot samples had to be eliminated during machine set up

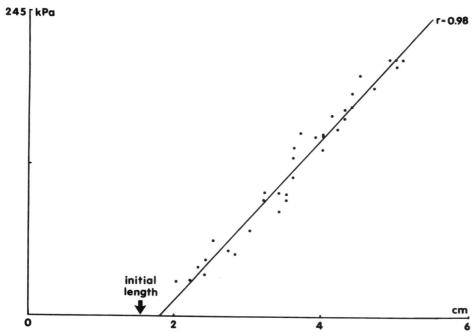

Fig. 1. Stress-strain diagram of PS coarse clot

surfaces, we observed a normal proliferation of fibroblasts. Mechanical disturbance of the clot surface greatly accelerated fibroblast proliferation, and the surface became completely covered with fibroblast growth (Fig. 2). HS clots treated in the same manner showed spheroidal deformation of cells, with no detectable proliferation (Fig. 3, Table 7).

The damage of cells on (nonwashed) HS clots was similar to the damage caused by the same sealant in liquid form, but the damaging effect occurred more slowly on the solid sealant.

Conductivity measurements on the supernatants of clot washings revealed the removal of more than 95% of salts contained in the clots after 4 washing cycles. Morphology and growth of fibroblasts were identical on washed and nonwashed PS clots, while the cytotoxicity of HS clots was reduced, but not completely eliminated, by extensive washing with isotonic NaCl solution (results not shown).

Table 6. Comparison of Fibrin Sealants

	PS	HS
Factor XIII (U/ml)	12.0	65.0
Conductivity (1:10 dilution with H$_2$O) (mS)	1.3	4.0
Osmolarity (mOsmol)	547.0	1 011.0

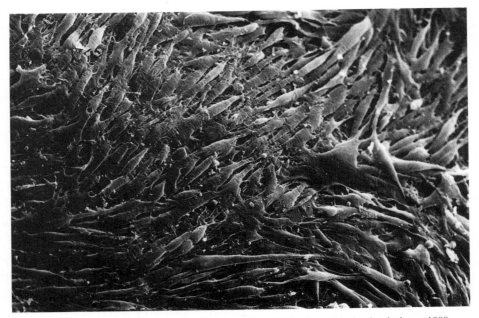

Fig. 2. Rich proliferation of fibroblasts on a cut PS clot. SEM, after critical point drying, x 1000

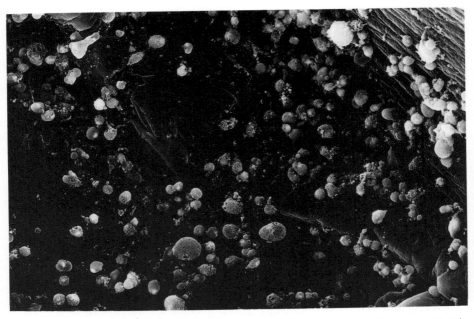

Fig. 3. Spheroidally deformed (damaged) fibroblasts on a HS fine clot after identical treatment as in Fig. 2

Table 7. Comparison of the Proliferation Rate of Fibroblasts (Cell Layer and Cell Suspension) when subjected to either PS or HS Sealer Protein Solution

	Photometric extinction at 570 nm		% Inhibition unphysiological –
	PS	HS	HS
Cell layer (mean of 3 diff. experiments ± SD)	.390±.130	.185±.077	53±3
cell suspension (mean of 3 diff. experiments ± SD)	.243±.190	.131±.112	67±7

Discussion

Because of the limited strength of Cryo and AF (Table 5), which results from a low clottable protein concentration (Table 3) and only ~ 35% α-chain crosslinking even after 2 hours (Table 4) no further experiments concerning histology and cell compatibility were carried out.

Fibrin sealant is a concentrated protein solution. Upon application, fibrinogen is coagulated by mixing with a thrombin-calcium chloride solution, following which the rigidity of the adhesives increases further as a result of fibrin crosslinking. The two preparations studied here produce clots with significantly different characteristics: PS clots are white (non-transparent) and of visco-elastic consistency, whereas HS clots are almost crystalclear and relatively brittle. Ferry and Morrisson [1] in 1947 described the formation of two different kinds of fibrin clots: white, non-transparent "coarse clots" formed at an ionic strength and pH value within the physiological range, and transparent "fine clots" produced at a higher ionic strength and/or pH value. Transition from one type to the other is smooth, with fibrinogen concentration, thrombin concentration, and reaction temperature as further influencing factors. In the present study, we determined electrical conductivity, osmolarity, and the kinetics of fibrin crosslinking of both sealants after adjustment of factor XIII content (Tables 4, 6). Micrographs of the fibrin clots produced were obtained under both light and scanning electron (SEM) microscopes and were compared with clots prepared from plasma and thrombin. Because HS differs from PS mainly by its high ionic strength outside the physiological range (causing the formation of almost amorphous clots), we examined the question of how the two sealants would differ in their influence on living cells. Considering the essential role of fibroblast proliferation in wound healing [7], we performed tests with human fibroblasts.

Our investigations were motivated by the striking differences in optical and mechanical properties between the two sealants after setting.

The essential difference between PS and HS is in ion content. PS conductivity is similar to that of isotonic saline solution, whereas HS conductivity is about three times greater.

Our results confirm the basic findings of Ferry and Morrison [1] that visco-elastic, nontransparent fibrin clots are formed at physiological ionic strength ("coarse" clots), whereas transparent, brittle "fine" clots are produced at a higher ionic strength. Our results indicate that this influence of ionic strength persists over a wide range of fibrinogen concentrations.

Clots produced from PS or plasma show similar fibrin characteristics, consisting of relatively thick, branching strands (Fig. 4); HS clots appear almost amorphous under identical conditions (Fig. 5). The porosity of HS (with 4 IU/ml thrombin) seen in Fig. 5 might be even less when applied in vivo (with 400–500 IU/ml thrombin) as it was found by Blombäck et al. [8] that increasing thrombin concentration results in reduced porosity of fibrin clots.

Both sealants are very similar in terms of fibrin crosslinking kinetics. Ionic strength above the physiological range is known to inhibit fibrin crosslinking [9]; therefore this anticipated effect was compensated for by adding factor XIII.

The significantly higher tensile strength in the coarse clots (PS) is similar to previous shear modulus data from Kanykowski et al. [10]. The elastic rigidity measurements of fine clots (HS) revealed less than one-tenth the shear modulus found for coarse clots. It is possible that the rigidity of the latter clots is primarily due to steric immobilization as has been suggested by Nelb et al. [11].

Because mechanical union is just one aspect of successful surgery, wound healing and hemostatic properties of the sealants must also be simultaneously evaluated.

The formation of fibrin and its crosslinking by factor XIIIa are essential for wound healing. The fibrin network produced under physiological conditions serves as a

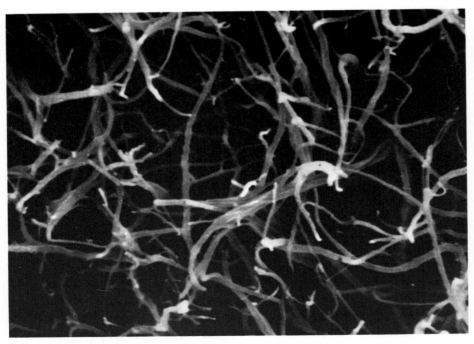

Fig. 4. Fibrin network in PS coarse clot very similar to plasma clot fibrin network. Scanning electron micrograph (SEM) after critical point drying.

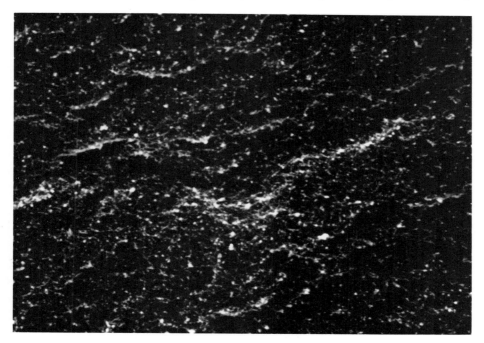

Fig. 5. Hardly detectable fibrin strands in a HS fine clot, conditions as in Fig. 4

matrix for the ingrowth of fibroblasts and the formation of collagen fibers [7, 12], thereby allowing for optimal wound healing. The formation of crosslinked fibrin is used not only for sealing tissues but for achieving hemostasis as well.

Up to now, many clinical and histologic reports [13, 14, 15, 16] describing satisfactory wound healing after fibrin sealant application have appeared. Thus the question arose whether the higher ion content of HS and the resulting altered fibrin structure of these clots influence fibroblast growth. Given the usual practice of mixing fibrin sealant with an equal volume of thrombin-CaCl$_2$ solution prior to application, we evaluated the influence of liquid sealants on fibroblasts after $1 + 1$ dilution with isotonic NaCl solution. We found that human fibroblasts were severely damaged within minutes by contact with liquid HS, whereas liquid PS does not cause any detectable damage, even after prolonged incubation (Figs. 6, 7). The cytotoxic effect of liquid HS, which is also demonstrated by its 50–60% inhibition of cell proliferation (Table 7), is most easily explained by its high ionic strength and osmolarity. Both HS clots (nonwashed) and liquid HS cause similar damage to cells, but cytotoxicity develops more slowly with the clots. This is understandable if we assume cytotoxicity to arise from soluble additives; the solution trapped in the clot and the cell medium applied take a certain time to equilibrate, by when the damaging additives are further diluted.

In order to distinguish whether the cytotoxity of HS clots is due to soluble substances trapped in the clot or to the altered fibrin structure, we washed PS and

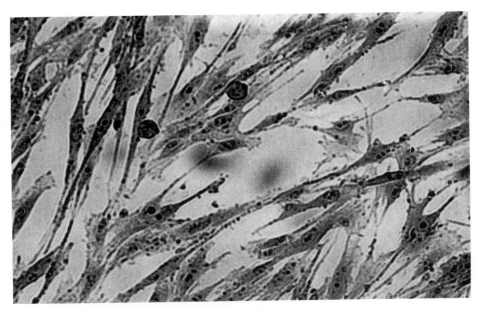

Fig. 6. Layer of fibroblasts 30 minutes after covering with PS, diluted 1 + 1. No detectable differences to controls. LM, carbol fuchsin staining, x 125

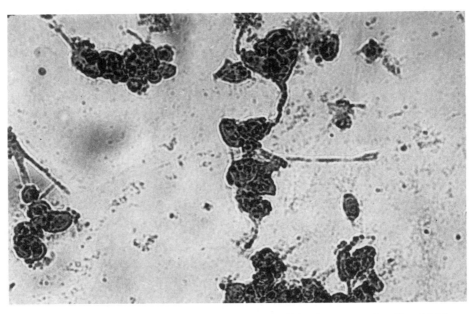

Fig. 7. Layer of fibroblasts 4 (!) minutes after covering with high salt concentration diluted 1 + 1. Damage to cell structure is clearly visible. Staining and enlargement as in Fig. 6

HS clots with isotonic NaCl solution. Conductivity measurements revealed that this procedure removed more than 95% of the conductive substances originally present in HS clots. Cells proliferated well on washed PS clots; washing reduced but did not eliminate cytotoxicity of HS clots [3].

Thus, the nearly absent structure of transparent fine clots appears to have a certain cytotoxic effect on fibroblasts in vitro. We consider this finding to have important implications in vivo. Although it may be assumed that the soluble components will diffuse out of a clot slowly, the typical "fine clot" structure will persist.

The importance of a stabilized fibrin network on fibroblast growth deserves special mention. The latter grow faster on cut PS clots than on the very smooth surfaces formed at the liquid-air interface of noncut clots. On the other hand, the same treatment on the cut surface did not improve fibroblast growth of washed HS concentration clots.

Beck et al. [17] in 1962 found that factor XIII is essential for normal fibroblast proliferation, they attributed the wound healing complications associated with factor XIII deficiency to a disturbance of fibroblast growth. These findings were later confirmed and extended by other investigators [18,19, 20]. According to Bruhn et al. [21], fibroblast proliferation is stimulated by the presence of factor XIII, whereas according to Kasai et al. [22], crosslinked fibrin rather than factor XIII is essential for the adherence of fibroblasts to the substrate and for well oriented cell growth. It was shown further that factor XIII itself may have an inhibitory effect on epidermal cell proliferation [23].

Our results indicate that crosslinked fibrin promotes attachment and growth of (human) fibroblasts only if present as PS coarse clots, whereas HS fine clots do not stimulate fibroblast proliferation and actually damage them, even at a comparable degree of crosslinking and after the additives that caused the formation of the fine clot structure have been removed.

Cryoprecipitate and glues from whole blood [2], carry other problems, such as poor standardization, lack of quality control, no virus inactivation, or little strength (e.g. AF, Table 5); the last point was corroborated by Hamm and Beer [24]. Other materials like COHN-fraction [24], though having good tensile strength, have very high viscosity as a major drawback.

It is obvious when comparing their different properties that synthetic sealants like acrylates [25] or gelatine-resorcin-formaldehyde [26, 27] have very limited applications.

References

1. Ferry JD, Morrison PR (1947) Preparation and properties of serum and plasma proteins. VIII. The conversion of human fibrinogen to fibrin under various conditions. J Amer Chem Soc 69:388–400.
2. Wolf G, Stammberger H (1984) Erste Berichte über die Anwendung eines autogenen Gewebeklebers in der Hals Nasen Ohrenheilkunde. HNO 32:1–4
3. Redl H, Schlag G, Dinges HP (1985) Vergleich zweier Fibrinkleber. Einfluß ionischer Zusätze auf Fibrinstruktur sowie Morphologie und Wachstum menschlicher Fibroblasten. Med Welt 36: 769–776

4. Redl H, Stank G, Hirschl A, Schlag G (1982) Fibrinkleber-Antibiotika-Gemische Festigkeit und Elutionsverhalten. In: Cotta H, Braun A (eds) Fibrinkleber in Orthopädie und Traumatologie. Thieme, Stuttgart, pp 178–181

5. Mosmann T (1983) Rapid colorimetric assay for cellular growth and survival: application to proliferation and cytotoxicity assays. J Immunol Methods 65:55–63

6. Bale MD, Müller MF, Ferry JD (1985) Rheological studies of creep and creep recovery of unligated fibrin clots: comparison of clots prepared with thrombin and ancord. Biopolymers 24: 461–482

7. Ross R (1968) The fibroblast and wound repair. Biol Rev 43:51–96

8. Blombäck B, Okada M, Forslind B, Larsson UT (1984) Fibrin gels as biological filters and interfaces. Biorheology 21:93–104

9. Seelich T, Redl HT (1980) Theoretische Grundlagen des Fibrinklebers. In: Schimpf K (ed) Fibrinogen, Fibrin und Fibrinkleber. F K Schattauer, Stuttgart, pp 199–208

10. Kamykowski GW, Mosher DF, Lorand L, Ferry JDT (1981) Modification of shear modulus and creep compliance of fibrin by fibronectin. Biophys Chem 13:25–28

11. Nelb GW, Gerth C, Ferry JD, Lorand L (1976) Biophys Chem 5:377

12. Beck E, Duckert F, Vogel A, Ernst M (1961) The influence of fibrin stabilizing factor on the growth of fibroblasts in vitro and wound healing. Thromb Diath Haemorrh 6:485–491

13. Spängler HP, Braun F (1983) Fibrinklebung in der operativen Medizin. Edition Medizin, Verlag Weinheim, Deerfield Beach, Florida, Basel

14. Scheele J (1984) Fibrinklebung. Springer-Verlag, Berlin, Heidelberg, New York

15. Köstering H, Kasten U, Artmann U, Ruskowski H, Beyer JM (1981) Behandlung von Hautnekrosen nach der Extravasation von Zytostatika mit Fibrinkleber. In: Blümel G, Haas S (eds) Mikrozirkulation und Prostaglandinstoffwechsel. Interaktion von Blutgerinnung und Fibrinolyse mit anderen proteolytischen Enzymsystemen. Neues über Fibrinogen, Fibrin und Fibrinkleber. Schattauerverlag, Stuttgart, pp 349–351

16. Rendl KH, Staindl O, Zelger J, Chmelizek-Feurstein CT (1980) Die Hauttransplantation mit Fibrinkleber beim Ulcus cruris. Akt Dermatol 6:199–203

17. Beck E, Duckert F, Vogel A, Ernst M (1962) Der Einfluß des fibrinstabilisierenden Faktors (FSF) auf Funktion und Morphologie von Fibroblasten in vitro. Z Zellforsch 57:327–346

18. Bruhn HD, Christopers E, Pohl J, Scholl G (1980) Regulation der Fibroblastenproliferierung durch Fibrinogen Fibrin, Fibronectin und Faktor XIII. In: Schimpf K (ed) Fibronogen, Fibrin und Fibrinkleber. F K Schattauer-Verlag, Stuttgart, pp 217–226

19. Turowski G, Schaadt M, Barthels M, Diehl V, Poliwada H (1980) Unterschiedlicher Einfluß von Fibrinogen und Faktor XIII auf das Wachstum von Primär- und Kulturfibroblasten. In: Schimpf K (ed) Fibrinogen, Fibrin und Fibrinkleber. F K Schattauer-Verlag, Stuttgart, pp 227–237

20. Knoche H, Schmitt G (1976) Autoradiographische Untersuchungen über den Einfluß des Faktors XIII auf die Wundheilung im Tierexperiment. Arzneimittelforsch – Drug Res 26:547–551

21. Bruhn HD, Pohl J (1981) Growth regulation of fibroblasts by thrombin, factor XIII and fibronectin. Klin Wochenschr 59:145–146

22. Kasai S, Kunimoto T, Nitta J (1983) Cross-linked of fibrin by activated factor XIII stimulated attachment, morphological changes and proliferation of fibroblasts. Biomed Res 4:155–160

23. Hashimoto T, Marks R (1984) Factor XIII inhibits epidermal cell migration in vitro. J Invest Dermatol 83:441–444

24. Hamm KD, Beer R (1985) Klebefestigkeitsuntersuchungen an biologischen Gewebeklebern. Z Exp Chir Transplant Künstliche Organe 18:281–288

25. Stoppa R, Henry X, Odimba E, Verhaeghe P, Largueche S, Myon Y (1980) Dacron tulle prosthesis and biological glue in the surgical treatment of incisional hernias. Nouv Presse Med 6:3541–3545

26. Vandor E, Jancsar L, Mozsary P, Reffy A, Demel Z (1980) Experience about the application of gelatin resorcinol formaldehyde tissue adhesive in experimental ruptured liver injury. Z Exp Chir Transplant Künstliche Organe 13:52–58

27. Bachet J, Gigou F, Laurian C, Bical O, Goudot B, Guilmet D (1981) 4-year clinical experience with the gelatin-resorcinol-formol biological glue in acute aortic dissection. J Thorac Cardiovasc Surg 83:212–217

Lysis and Absorption of Fibrin Sealant (Tissucol/Tisseel)

(In Vitro and In Vivo Experiments)

H. Pflüger

Key words: Fibrin, wound repair, fibrinolysis, ^{125}I-elimination

Abstract

In order to determine the optimal fibrin thrombin adhesive system (FTAS) composition for resistance to fibrinolysis, in vivo lysis was tested by adding increasing amounts of the fibrinolysis inhibitor aprotinin to ^{125}I-FS; urokinase and plasminogen were administered in vitro while measuring protein and iodine[125] release. The correlation between protein and iodine[125] release clearly reflects the interdependence of these parameters; disjunction of radioactivity from the protein molecule was ruled out. In vitro, fibrinolysis is inhibited to a nearly unlimited extent by aprotinin. In vivo, aprotinin improves fibrinolysis inhibition only up to a maximum of 1500 KIU/ml clot, thereby significantly altering the maximum elimination of [125]iodine and FS half-life as well. Higher doses of aprotinin applied in vivo remain without effect upon FS stability. In human surgery, the addition of aprotinin to FS is recommended for strictly hemostatic application only, not for tissue synthesis such as nerve and microvessel anastomoses in plastic reconstructive surgery.

The aim of the second study was to investigate the degradation of fibrinogen thrombin adhesive system (FTAS) and the process of wound healing after partial kidney resection in rats using FTAS for induction of local hemostasis. In 28 rats partial kidney resection was performed bilaterally. Hemostasis was achieved with FTAS. Four experimental groups were formed. Group F ($n = 3$): hemostasis with unlabeled FTAS, subcutaneous injection of 0.1 ml = 60 µCi Na [125]I. Group G ($n = 3$): hemostasis with unlabeled FTAS, subcutaneous injection of 0.1 ml = 60 µCi ^{125}I-labeled FTAS, Group H ($n = 6$): hemostasis with ^{125}I-labeled FTAS. Group I ($n = 16$): treated like group H. In groups F–H ^{125}I elimination in 24-h urine samples was determined with a gamma-scintillation counter. Pairs of animals in group I were killed after 2, 6, 12, and 24 h and 3, 7, 14, and 21 days.

Kidneys were examined under the light and electron microscope and by autoradiography. In animals of groups G and H two peaks of ^{125}I excretion were observed: one peak within the first 48 h postoperatively which corresponded to the amount of free iodine injected with FTAS (FTAS contains 15% free iodine) and a second peak after 120 h which was most probably due to the degradation of FTAS. Fibrinolysis was not observed. FTAS was resorbed mainly by macrophages. The time course of wound healing paralleled that of physiological fibrinogen concentration. Renal parenchymal damage was not observed.

Introduction

Fibrin plays a central role in the physiological process of wound healing. According to examinations by Key [8] fibrin induces the chemotaxis of polymorphonuclear granulocytes and introduces the initial inflammatory phase of the healing process. There is no doubt that the concentration of fibrin and the platelet content of the thrombus as well as a variety of other factors are in direct interaction and influence the duration of the healing process.

Use of Tissucol, a sealing method that has been employed for years, imitates the physiological process, applying unphysiologically high concentrations of fibrinogen. The influence of the artificial clot on chemotaxis and the resulting induction of macrophages and fibroblasts and of collagen fiber formation is unknown. Other unanswered questions are

a) the importance of the local potential of the sealed tissue for lysis and degradation of the fibrin clot and

b) the necessity of adding fibrinolysis inhibitors to the film clots and their appropiate concentrations. It was the objective of the experiments described below to test the fibrinolysis of a Tissucol clot in vitro with and without proteinase inhibitors, and to obtain further results on cellular fibrin degradation in in vivo experiments.

First Study

Materials and Methods

In Vitro Experiment

0.1 ml ^{125}I-FS Human Immuno (60 µCi/0.1 ml) was clotted by adding 0.1 ml thrombin (4 NIH-U/ml) and $CaCl_2$ (0.04 M/Liter) and incubated for 30 min at 37°C. Aprotinin (5000 KIU/ml clot) was added to series A. There was no aprotinin in series B.

In vitro lysis of FTAS was performed by layers of 1 ml urokinase (5.25 Plough-U/ml) and 1 ml plasminogen solution (0.2 CTU/ml) at 37°C permanent incubation. The supernatant was exchanged every 12 h. Protein content was established photometrically at an extinction of 280 nm, and the content of ^{125}I was measured by a gamma-scintillation counter.

In Vivo Experiment

Twenty-one albino rats (Wistar) with an average weight of 320 g were used as test animals. The animals were kept in single metabolite cages and fed with Tagger whole food and water ad libitum. In order to avoid any intermediary retention of ^{125}I in the thyroid gland, the animals were given 25 drops of Lugol's solution (ÖAB 9, solutio jodi aquosi) in 40 ml drinking water 3 days before the tests were started. In Ketalar (60 mg/kg body weight) and Rompun (8 mg/kg body weight) general anesthesia, two skin pockets of 1.5×0.5 were formed on the back of the animals and 0.2 ml FTAS was injected into these pockets.

Fibrin sealant:

0.1 ml ^{125}I-FS human Immuno (60 µCi/0.1 ml)

0.1 ml thrombin (4 NIH-U/ml)

CaCl$_2$ 0.04 M/liter

Group C ($n = 7$) was treated without aprotinin, while in group D ($n = 7$) 1500 KIU/ml clot and in group E $n = 7$) 5000 KIU/ml clot were added to the FTAS. In animals of group C–E ^{125}I elimination was counted by gamma-scintillation counter in urine collected over 24 h until the 7th day after surgery.

All the results were indicated as mean value with standard deviation.

Results

In Vitro Experiment

The correlation coefficient of protein concentration (extinction at 280 nm) and radioactivity counted was $r = 0.97$ for both series A and series B. Regression line $y = 0.02 \times + 0.04$ (Fig. 1).

The samples with aprotinin (series A) showed slow fibrinolysis. A maximum of 5% of the total activity was absorbed per 12 h and the stability of the clot lasted for more than a week. In the samples without aprotinin (series B) the maximum degradation was found after 36 h, 40% of the total activity being released (Fig. 2). After 60 h the whole FS clot was dissolved.

In Vivo Experiment

All the animals survived the surgical intervention and the observation period of 7 days.

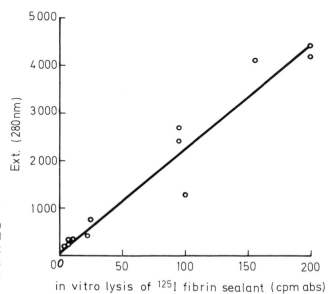

Fig. 1. Correlation of protein concentration and counted radioactivity. Measurement every 12 hours after lysis of a I^{125} fibrin sealant clot with urokinase-plasminogen

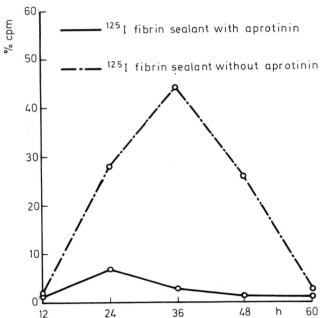

Fig. 2. Fibrinolysis expressed in radioactivity counted in 12 h urine samples of rats

The maximum ^{125}I excretion in animals of group C was found after 1.75 ± 0.5 days, in group D (1500 KIU/ml clot) after 3.2 ± 0.45 days, and in group E after 3.5 ± 1.29 days.

Statistical evaluation of the results by means of the hour t-test showed a significant time difference in the elimination maximum ($p<0.01$) between animals of groups C and D, and C and E. Comparison of the groups D (1500 KIU/ml) and E (5000 KIU/ml) showed no significant time difference in the ^{125}I excretion maximum. (Fig. 3) shows mean values of ^{125}I elimination as a percentage of the total dose applied in

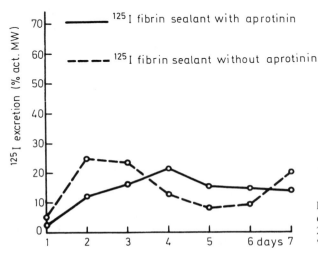

Fig. 3. Mean values and standard deviation of I^{125} excretion in 24 h urine samples, expressed in % of total radioactivity applied

animals of groups C and D during an observation period of 7 days. In animals of group C we found a two-stage course of the graph: A first elimination peak occurred after 2 days ($\bar{x}\sim24\%$); ^{125}I excretion then reached a minimum on the 5th day after surgery ($\bar{x}\sim8\%$) but a further increase was observed on the 7th day after surgery ($\bar{x}\sim20\%$). In animals of group D this two-stage course of the graph could not be observed. They showed a slow increase in ^{125}I excretion, the peak being on the 4th day after surgery ($\bar{x}\sim21\%$), as well as a slow decrease in ^{125}I excretion. On the 7th day after surgery 14% of the total dose applied was eliminated. ^{125}I elimination in animals of group E was almost identical to that in animals of group D.

FS Half-life

The Half-life (period of time after which half of the iodine dose applied has been eliminated) was 2.16 ± 0.13 days in animals of group C, 2.82 ± 0.31 days in group D, and 2.92 ± 0.25 days in group E. There was a statistically significant difference ($P < 0.01$) between animals of groups C and D, and groups C and E. There was no statistically important difference between groups D and E.

Second Study

Materials and Methods

In the second study we examined the degradation of fibrinogen thrombin adhesive system (FTAS) during healing after partial kidney resection in rats, using FTAS for production of local hemostasis. We followed the fate of the autologous fibrin clot histologically and by monitoring the redistribution of ^{125} iodinated fibrin fragments.

FTAS was applied on a supporting collagen fleece (Disperger, Vienna), placed on the resection wound [12], and lightly pressed digitally on to the resection area for 60 s. Twenty-eight male albino rats were used (Wistar SPF breed, average weight 350 g). The animals were kept in single cages and fed with Tagger complete food and water ad libitum. In order to achieve complete blockage of iodine absorption into the thyroid gland, all animals were given 25 drops of Lugol's solution (ÖAB 9, solutio jodi aquosi) in 40 ml drinking water 5 days before starting the experiment. Under diethyl ether anesthesia the kidneys were exposed through lumbar incisions, bilateral lower partial kidney resections were performed, and hemostasis of the parenchymatous wound was achieved with FTAS as described above. Twenty percent of the renal parenchyma was removed. The 28 animals were divided into four experimental groups:

Group F (n = 3): Bilateral partial kidney resection, hemostasis with unlabeled FTAS, subcutaneous injection of 0.1 ml = 60 µCi Na ^{125}I (Amersham, IMS, 1 P ^{125}I sodium thiosulfate).

Group G (n = 3): Bilateral partial resection, hemostasis with unlabeled FTAS, subcutaneous injection of 0.1 ml = 60 µCi ^{125}I-FTAS.

Group H (n = 6): Bilateral partial kidney resection, hemostasis with ^{125}I-FTAS.

Group I (n = 16): Bilateral partial kidney resection, hemostasis with ^{125}I-FTAS.

The ^{125}I-elimination in a 24-h urine sample from animals in groups F–H was measured by a gamma-scintillation counter daily up to the 10th postoperative day.

For morphological studies pairs of animals of group I underwent laparotomy 2, 6, 12, and 24 h and 3, 7, 14, and 21 days after surgery. The kidneys which had been partially resected were perfused with Hanks' solution to remove all intrarenal blood and then perfused for 10 min with 2.5% glutaraldehyde in 0.1 M cacodylate buffer (pH 7.4) [9]. The tissue samples were embedded in Epon 812 and 1-μ m sections were stained with 1% toluidine blue. For autoradiography Kodak Nuclear Track-Emulsion was applied to the sections, the exposure time being 28 days at 4°C. Ultrathin sections were examined in an EM9S electron microscope.

Serum creatinine and BUN were determined photometrically on the 3rd and 10th postoperative days.

Results

General

No animal died immediately after operation or within the period of observation. Three animals developed a unilateral wedge-shaped, ischemic renal infarction. Parenchymatous destruction to a maximum depth of 3–20 tubular lumina could be found in all other kidneys. In two cases a stone was found in the renal pelvis. Diffractometric X-ray analysis showed the stone composition to be calcium oxalate monohydrate. No animal developed uremia.

Dynamics of ^{125}Iodinated FTAS and ^{125}I Sodium Thiosulfate

Mean values and standard deviations of the ^{125}I excretion in 24-h urine samples indicated as a percentage of the ^{125}I total excretion during the 10-day observation period for animals of groups F–H are shown in Fig. 4.

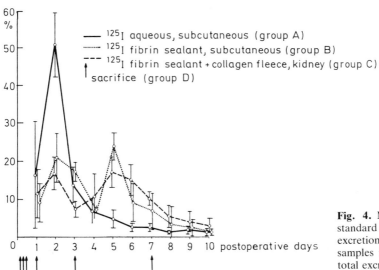

Fig. 4. Mean values and standard deviation of I^{125} excretion in 24 h urine samples indicated in % of total excretion per 10 days

Group F (Subcutaneous Injection of 60 µCi Na ^{125}I)

^{125}I excretion was maximal on the 2nd postoperative day (50.5 ± 8.4%) and an exponential decrease of ^{125}I elimination occurred after this time. By the 3rd postoperative day 80% of the measured total dose had been eliminated. ^{125}I elimination on the 10th postoperative day was 1.5 ± 0.75%.

Group G [Subcutaneous Injection of 0.1 ml (Containing Approximately 75 mg Protein) = 60 µCi FTAS]

Maximal ^{125}I excretion occurred on the 2nd (20.6 ± 6.2%) and 5th postoperative days (23.6% ± 3.5%). The least ^{125}I elimination occurred during the 4th postoperative day (7% ± 1.3%). A slow decrease in ^{125}I elimination occurred from the 5th postoperative day onwards. ^{125}I excretion on the 10th postoperative day was 1.1% ± 0.6% of the measured total dose.

Group H ^{125}I-FTAS for Hemostasis of Kidney Wounds

Maximal ^{125}I elimination occurred on the 2nd (16.5% ± 4.2%) and 5th postoperative days (16.5% ± 3.8%). The lowest excretion rate occurred on the 3rd postoperative day (7.3% ± 2%). A slow decrease in ^{125}I elimination occurred after the 5th postoperative day. ^{125}I elimination on the 10th postoperative day was 3% ± 2% of the measured total dose excreted.

Radioisotope excretion did not depend on the daily volume of urine.

Histological, Electron Microscopic, and Autoradiographic Findings in Animals of Group I

2, 6, and 12 Hours After Operation. No reaction of connective tissue was observed under the light or on the electron microscope. Collagen fleece was inhibited with erythrocytes and partly lifted off the parenchymatous area by small hematomas.

24 Hours After Operation. Light and electron microscope studies showed emigration of neutrophilic granulocytes and macrophages into the intersticium (Fig. 5). Autoradiography showed larger amounts of labeled fibrin at the area of adhesion.

3 Days After Operation. Cell-rich granulation tissue and infiltration of granulocytes was seen under the light microscope (Fig. 6). Marked resorption of fibrin clots by phagocytosing macrophages (Figs. 7, 8), as well as capillary outgrowth, was seen under the electron microscope. A high concentration of radioactively labeled FTAS was still present.

7 Days After Operation. Collagen fiber appeared and isolated remnants of radioactively labeled fibrin were seen in the granulation tissue with numerous macrophages.

14 and 21 Days After Operation. Collagen-rich granulation tissue with a markedly decreased number of infiltrating cells was found. Until the 14th postoperative day,

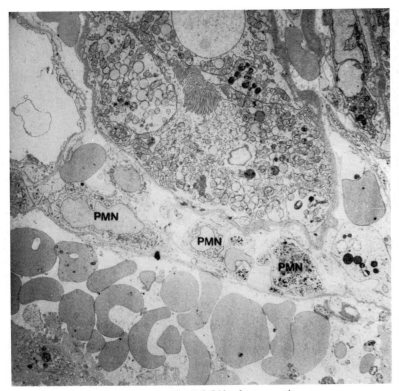

Fig. 5. Immigration of leucocytes (PMN) 24 h after operation

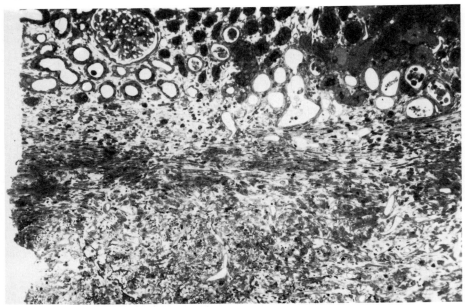

Fig. 6. Cell rich granulation tissue and leucocytes 3 days after operation (× 32)

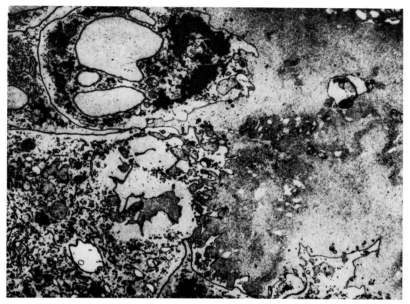

Fig. 7. FTAS resorption by macrophages 3rd postoperative day (× 5700)

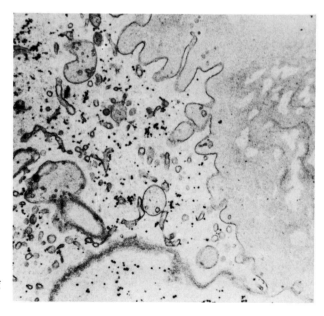

Fig. 8. Partial enlargement of Fig. 7 (× 27000)

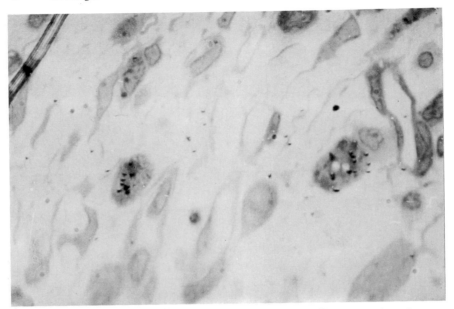

Fig. 9. Macrophages with incorporated degradation products of I^{125} labeled fibrin sealant

radioactively labeled fibrin was found in macrophages (Fig. 9). There was decreasing infiltration of round cells.

Discussion

Urokinase plasminogen-induced in vitro lysis of ^{125}I-labeled fibrin sealant shows an excellent correlation of both measuring parameters after measuring protein content and released radioactivity. This seems to prove that in vitro ^{125}I is not balanced out and washed off by protein molecules. It has to be presumed that measurements of ^{125}I excretion in 24-h urine in vivo are directly proportional to clot degradation.

In vitro the resistance of FS to urokinase plasminogen-induced lysis may be increased most efficiently and for as long as is wanted by the addition of aprotinin [6,11]. Measurement of ^{125}I activity released in series A and B supports these findings. As expected, the in vivo experiment showed that FTAS with aprotinin (1500 KIU/ml clot) is more resistant to fibrinolysis than FTAS without aprotinin. Increasing the aprotinin concentration to 5000 KIU/ml clot does not cause a delay in the ^{125}I elimination maximum nor any prolongation of the biological half-life. This seems to prove that aprotinin (1500 KIU/ml clot) is sufficient for stopping local fibrinolytic activity, and that the physiological degradation of FTAS by phagocytosis cannot be influenced by aprotinin.

^{125}I is mostly excreted in the urine after absorption of labeled iodine into the thyroid gland has been prevented by prior oral administration of an overdose of stable iodine. Analogous to the in vivo examinations by Alkjaersig [1] and Dudock

[4, 5] the determination of ^{125}I elimination in urine provides information about the degradation of labeled fibrin clots.

After subcutaneous injection, ^{125}I sodium thiosulfate was eliminated in the urine maximally on the 2nd postoperative day (50.5% ± 8.4% of total elimination per 10 days) in a single peak, reflecting the elimination pattern of free ^{125}I sodium thiosulfate. By contrast, after subcutaneous injection of ^{125}I-FTAS (Group G) and also after application of ^{125}I-FTAS in a collagen fleece directly to the renal parenchyma (group H) there were two peaks of ^{125}I excretion, one on the 2nd and one on the 5th postoperative day. The first peak after 2 days corresponded with the maximal excretion of unbound iodine in FTAS, which consisted of about 15% of the total applied radioactivity. (The TCA precipitable radioactivity of labeled charges of FTAS amounted to an average of 85%.) The operation itself may have delayed the maximum excretion of free, non-protein-bound iodine to the 2nd postoperative day.

The second peak of ^{125}I excretion between the 3rd and 5th postoperative days in animals of groups G and H coincided with the resorption of the fibrin clot by macrophages (group I) (Fig. 5) and may thus be derived from small iodinated fibrin fragments or from iodine freed in the process of clot organization. These data suggest that the fibrin clot was not dissolved until the 3rd day and could therefore provide hemostasis during this critical time. The protracted secretion of radioactivity after the 5th postoperative day in animals of group H may be caused by slow release of fibrinolytic fragments from macrophages (Fig. 6). We excluded the possibility that the collagen fleece interfered with the resorption of FTAS by finding that urinary iodine excretion was identical in groups G and H.

Wound healing after clot formation is initiated by emigration of granulocytes, macrophages and by capillary sprouting. (The Importance of Fibrin in Wound Repair, see G. Schlag et al.). Bösch [2] claimed that FTAS on a porous carrier accelerated wound healing in bone when compared with controls in which FTAS had not been used. Since proper controls for our kidney resections could not be obtained – because the untreated kidney wound would cause recurrent severe hemorrhage [3] and because mechanical damage of the kidney tissue may also cause conditions different from those caused by surgical treatment – no conclusions concerning the speed of wound healing in our experimental system could be drawn. In addition cyanoacrylate tissue adhesive cannot be used as a control because of its cytotoxic activity. The results of wound healing in rats after partial kidney resection and application of FTAS are similar to studies of wound healing in the rabbit's ear with physiological fibrin concentrations [7]. The use of homologous fibrinogen cryopreci-pitate excluded any possible influence of foreign protein on hemostasis. Eosinophilic infiltration as a sign of allergic reaction [10] was not observed.

The wedge-shaped ischemic necroses (3/32) were due to the division at operation of a functional end-artery.

Comparing the results of the in vivo experiments with the data on the physiological wound healing process contained in the chapter "The Importance of Fibrin in Wound Repair" by G. Schlag et al., we find absolute agreement between the physiological process and the application of Tissucol as regards the time of wound healing, the inflammatory phase, and fibroplasia. The highly concentrated fibrin clot with addition of proteinase inhibitors in no way impedes the influx of polymorpho-nuclear granulocytes and macrophages and thus cellular fibrin degradation. Connective tissue proliferation and formation of granulation tissue are not influenced either. The excessive increase of proteinase inhibitor concentrations in the clot prevents the urokinase plasminogen-induced lysis of the fibrin clot in the in vitro test, although only a short-term delay in cellular degradation by proteinase inhibitors up to a maximum concentration of 1500 KIU aprotinin is possible. Taking into consideration that even short-term prolongation of fibrin stability induces increased influx of macrophages and thus fibroblasts and collagen fibers, it should be a clinical consequence of this examination to vary the addition of fibrinolysis inhibitors according to the clinical field of application of the fibrin sealant.

If atraumatic tissue synthesis has priority, such as in microvascular anastomoses and nerve anastomoses, no aprotinin should be added, thus avoiding unnecessary connective tissue proliferation, collagen fiber formation, and shrinking cicatrization. Sealing of parenchymatous organs such as the kidney, liver, and spleen certainly requires safe long-term hemostasis, justifying the application of aprotinin (1500 KIU/ml clot) in the fibrin clot.

References

1. Alkjaersing N, Fletscher AP, Sherry S (1959) The mechanism of clot dissolution by plasmin. Journal of Clinical Investigation 38, 1068
2. Bösch P, Braun F, Eschberger J, Kovac W, Spängler HP (1977) The action of high-concentrated fibrin on one healing. Archiv für Orthopädie und Unfallchirurgie 89, 259
3. Braun F, Henning K, Holle J, Kovac W, Rauchenwald K, Spängler HP, Urlesberger H (1977) A biological adhesive system (Fibrin) in partial kidney resection. Zentralblatt für Chirurgie 102, 1235
4. Dudock de Wit C, Krijinen HW, den Ottolander GJH (1962) The measurement of fibrinolytic activity with I^{131}-labeled clots I. The methods. Thrombosis and Haemostatis (Stuttgart) 8, 315
5. Dudock de Wit C, Krijinen HW, den Ottolander GJH (1972) The measurement of fibrinolytic activity with ^{131}I-labeled clots II. Application. Thrombosis and Haemostatis (Stuttgart) 8, 322
6. Guttmann J (1978) Untersuchungen eines Fibrinklebers für die Anwendung in der Chirurgie peripherer Nerven. Diplomarbeit, Inst f Botanik, Techn Mikroskopie und Organ Rohstofflehre. Techn Univ Wien
7. Jennings MA, Florey HW (1970) Healing. In: General pathology. Florey L (ed.), Chapter 17, p. 480. Oxford: Lloyd-Luces
8. Kay AB, Pepper DS, Ewart MR (1973)Generation of chemotactic activity for leukocytes by the action of thrombin on human fibrinogen. Nature 243:56–57
9. Maunsbach AB (1966) The influence of different fixatives and fixation methods on the ultrastructure of rat kidney proximal tubule cells. I. Comparison of different perfusion fixation methods and of gluteraldehyde, formaldehyde and osmium tetroxide fixatives. Journal of Ultrastructure Research 15, 242
10. Pflüger H, Lunglmayr G, Breitenecker G (1976) Anastomosis of the vas deferense employing concentrated fibrinogen: a experimental study in rabbits. Wiener klinische Wochenschrift 88, 24, 800
11. Redl H, Schlag G, Dinges H, Kuderna H, Seelich T (1982) Background and methods of "fibrin sealing". In: Biomaterials (Winter D, Gibbons DF, Plenk H – eds.), John Wiley and Sons, Ltd. Chichester, 669–676
12. Spängler HP (1978) Tissue adhesion and local hemostasis using fibrinogen, thrombin and clotring factor XIII. (Experimental investigation – Clinical experience) Wiener klinische Wochenschrift 88, Suppl 49

Preliminary Results of a Randomized Controlled Study on the Risk of Hepatitis Transmission of a Two-Component Fibrin Sealant (Tissucol/Tisseel)

G. Eder, M. Neumann, R. Cerwenka, and K. Baumgarten

Key words: two-component fibrin sealant, hepatitis, ALT, gamma-GT, cerclage, conization

Abstract

A hundred patients who were to undergo cerclage or conization were entered into the study, being assigned to either group A or B on a random basis, irrespective of the type of surgery planned. Group A received conventional surgery plus two-component fibrin sealant, group B received conventional surgery alone.

The objectives of the study were to demonstrate the efficacy of fibrin sealant as a sealing adjunct in cerclage and as an aid to wound healing in conization. A further objective was to evaluate the risk of hepatitis B and hepatitis non-A/non-B transmission through fibrin sealant. Efficacy results are published elsewhere; here data are presented only on the risk of viral hepatitis transmission.

Of the 100 patients who had entered the study, 69 had a sufficient number of blood samples taken to qualify for evaluation of the hepatitis risk (group A: n = 31; group B: n = 38). None of the patients in either group contracted hepatitis B or non-A/non-B.

Introduction

Tisseel or Tissucol is a biological two-component fibrin sealant which is used to achieve hemostasis, to seal leakages, to glue tissue, or to support sutures. Tisseel has been found also to enhance wound healing [1]. The freeze-dried product is manufactured from pooled plasma of selected donors. Donors of this plasma are tested at every donation for HBs antigenemia using radioimmunoassay. To reduce the risk of nonA/non-B hepatitis transmission [2, 3, 4], only plasma of alanine aminotransferase (ALT) levels below 25 U/liter (reaction temperature 25°C, optimized method; [5] are used for manufacturing fibrin sealant. Thus far, two prospective, nonrandomized studies have been published investigating the risk of hepatitis transmission associated with the use of fibrin sealant. One such study was conducted in general surgery [6], the other in ENT surgery [7]. In neither of the two studies has a case of hepatitis B been seen that might have been attributable to the use of fibrin sealant. In a substudy to the ENT study, two groups of ten patients each were also tested for transaminase at biweekly intervals for a total period of 8 months. In none of these patients could an increase in ALT beyond 50 U/liter be seen.

The study which is described below was a prospective, randomized, controlled study investigating the efficacy of fibrin sealant as an adjunct to conventional surgical techniques employed for cerclage and conization in obstetrics and gynecology, respectively. In its context patients were monitored for potential virus hepatitis associated with its use.

Material and Methods

Patient Group Assignment Procedure

Patients were assigned to group A or B by computer random numbers, irrespective of whether they were to undergo cerclage or conization. Patients in group A received two-component fibrin sealant in addition to conventional surgical methods; patients in group B served as a control and received conventional surgical treatment only. Cerclage was performed around the 16th week of pregnancy.

When patients were entered, they received envelopes bearing consecutive numbers which assigned them to either group A or B. This made it impossible for the surgeon to give preference to one of the two methods (conventional surgery alone or conventional surgery plus fibrin sealant). Each patient consented to entering the study in writing.

Dosage

All patients in group A were treated with 1 ml of fibrin sealant, which corresponds to approx. 100 mg fibrinogen. One lot of product was used.

Laboratory Tests for Viral Hepatitis

Blood samples were taken immediately before surgery, on the 3rd, 7th, and 14th days postsurgery, and 4, 6, 8, 10, 12 and 24 weeks postsurgery. Shorter intervals, it was felt, would have led to poor patient compliance. From each sample of whole blood, serum was obtained by routine hospital methods. Two milliliters of each serum sample was deep-frozen to provide documentation samples and the rest was tested for ALT, γ-GT, HBsAg, and HBsAb. If a sample proved positive for HBsAg or HBsAb, further tests were done to clarify the patient status, including tests for HBcAb, HBeAg, and HBeAb.

ALT was determined using commercially available reagent kits (Boehringer Mannheim; GPT optimized) at a reaction temperature of 25°C (recommendation of the German Society for Clinical Chemistry) [5]. For internal quality control three commercially available control sera were used (Monitrol I and II, Merz and Dade; and Precinorm U, Boehringer Mannheim) along with an in-house serum. The controls were tested at the beginning and end of each test series. Kinetics were measured using a Beckman spectral photometer (Model 25) and printer. Samples were measured manually and extinctions were printed at 60s. intervals. Extinction differences per minute ($\triangle$ U/min) were converted into U/liter using an extinction coefficient of 1756. Measuring time: 3 min; wavelength: Hg 365 nm. The manufacturer defines the normal range for women to be $\leq$ 17 U/liter [8, 9].

γ-GT was determined using commercially available kits by Boehringer Mannheim (Monotest Gamma-GT new) [10]. Reaction temperature: 25°C; measuring time: 3 min; print out of extinctions every 60 s.; wavelength: Hg 405 nm. Extinction differences ($\triangle$ U/min) were converted into U/liter using an extinction coefficient of 1158. The manufacturer defines the normal range for women as between 4 and 18 U/liter [11]. The internal quality control of γ-GT was performed in analogy to ALT determination.

HBsAg and HBsAb were determined using RIA-QUICK (Immuno AG, Vienna), AUSRIA, and AUSAB (Abbott). Determination of HBcAb, HBeAg and HBeAb was performed using CORZYME and HBe-EIA (ELISA Method, Abbott). Four in-house quality control sera which were calibrated against international standards were used to determine HBsAg and HBsAb. For HBsAg determination the internal quality control sera were calibrated against the HBs Reference Antigen (subtypes *ad* and *ay*) of the Paul-Ehrlich-Institute, Frankfurt/Main (concentration 50 000 U/ml), and the British Reference Preparation of Hepatitis B Surface Antigen (1st British Reference Preparation established 1982 – concentration 100 Units by definition) [12]. The limit of detection for HBsAg was also tested using the standard of the Paul-Ehrlich-Institute and was found to be 0.5 ng of HBsAg/ml. For quality control of HBsAb determination the HBV-Referenzserum (IgG) of the Paul-Ehrlich-Institute Frankfurt/Main was used in a concentration of 25 IU/vial and the WHO Anti-Hepatitis B Immunoglobulin Standard, 1st Reference Preparation 1977, lot 26.1.77, in a concentration of 50 IU anti-hepatitis B immune globulin [13, 16]. HBsAg-positive results were confirmed using the inhibition test in the radioimmunoassay. HBsAb-positive findings having a concentration of $\leq$ 10 mU/ml were considered negative.

Results

Altogether 100 patients (group A, $n = 50$; group B, $n = 50$) were recruited into the study; 72 underwent cerclage, 28 conization (Table 1).

An evaluation of the efficacy of fibrin sealant in the treatment of cerclage and conization has been published elsewhere. In the following only the hepatitis risk associated with fibrin sealant is discussed. To evaluate this risk, only patients were

Table 1. Patient sample and group assignment

Group	Treatment	n
A (with Fibrin Sealant)	Cerclage	37
A (with Fibrin Sealant)	Conization	13
B (without Fibrin Sealant)	Cerclage	35
B (without Fibrin Sealant)	Conization	15
	Total	100

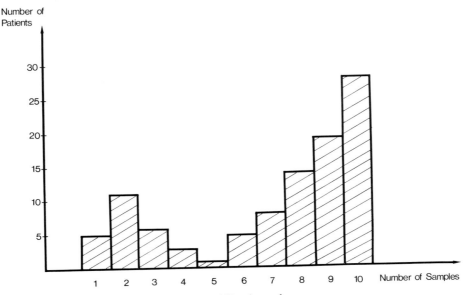

Fig. 1. Frequency distribution of patients and blood samples

used from whom at least seven consecutive blood samples (over a period of at least 10 weeks postsurgery) were available. Of the 100 patients in the study only 69 presented for blood sampling seven times or more (Fig. 1). Table 2 gives the proportion of patients who had at least seven blood samples taken and qualified for evaluation of the hepatitis risk and those who did not. As can be seen, 31 patients (23 cerclage and 8 conization) qualified in group A and 38 patients (29 cerclage and 9 conization) in group B. The percentage of patients undergoing conization in groups A and B was about the same (62% and 60%, resp.). In group B the percentage of patients undergoing cerclage (83%) was higher than in group A (62%).

Table 2. Proportions of patients qualifying and not qualifying for the evaluation of hepatitis transmission

	Nonevaluable patients	Evaluable patients	Sum (100%)
A/cerclage	14 (38%)	23 (62%)	37
A/conization	5 (38%)	8 (62%)	13
B/cerclage	6 (17%)	29 (83%)	35
B/conization	6 (40%)	9 (60%)	15
Total	31	69	100

Hepatitis B Markers

From among the 69 patients who had at least seven consecutive blood samples taken, one had to be excluded from evaluation because of receiving hepatitis B vaccination in the 4th, 8th and 12th week post fibrin sealant application.

Of the remaining 68 patients, two tested positive for HBsAb of all blood samples taken, including the preoperative one. These patients must be considered immune to hepatitis B. In three more patients HBsAb was detected on the 2nd and 7th postoperative days in concentrations below 15 mU/ml. Two of these three patients tested negative for HBsAb on all other blood samples. In one patient in group B who underwent cerclage, HBsAb findings were positive, in a concentration of as low as 13 mU/ml 6 months postsurgery. Two of the patients tested positive for HBsAg on all samples, including the preoperative sample.

Hepatitis Non-A/Non-B Markers

By definition, non-A/non-B hepatitis can only be suspected if ALT is increased postoperatively to 2.5 times the upper limit of normal. In all, 12 ALT increases (ALT > 20 U/liter) were detected, eight in group A and four in group B. Two patients (both in group B) only had slightly increased values initially (in one case 39 U/liter preoperatively, followed by normal findings on all postoperative samples; in another case a pathological 49 U/liter on the preoperative sample, which normalized in the course of the subsequent 2 weeks). Two more patients in group B had slightly increased ALT values without hepatitis B markers 6 months postoperatively (41 and 46 U/liter). One patient in each group had increased ALT values in postoperative weeks 6 and 8 (46 and 40 U/liter, resp.) without hepatitis B markers. None of the patients had clinical symptoms of non-A/non-B hepatitis.

In addition to ALT, γ-GT was monitored as an indicator of the possible presence of non-A/non-B hepatitis. Nine increased γ-GT values were found in all (six in group A, three in group B). The increased γ-GT results were often borderline. One patient in each group had preoperatively increased γ-GT (114 and 41 U/liter, resp.) which returned to normal in the course of the observation period in one patient and dropped to half the initial value in the other. One more patient in group A had a one-time increase in γ-GT of 46 U/liter 10 weeks postoperatively.

Discussion

The main ingredient of two-component fibrin sealant is fibrinogen, which is present in a concentration ranging from 70 to 110 mg/ml. Products made from human plasma are known to have the potential of transmitting viral hepatitis, unless special donor screening methods are used and/or products are subjected to a virus inactivation procedure. To exclude hepatitis B, donations have been tested for HBsAg before such plasma is used for processing into plasma derivatives ever since third generation test methods became available (radioimmunoassy and/or ELISA). This measure dramatically reduced hepatitis B transmission. Nevertheless, a high percentage (up to 98%) of hemophiliacs have been shown to have hepatitis B markers [14]. In addition, chimpanzee trials have shown that infectivity of some plasmas persists despite negative HBsAg findings in the radioimmunoassay, rendering hepatitis B transmission possible [15].

The difference between the infection titer and HBsAg titer in the radioimmunoassay may be as large as two or three orders of magnitude. This means that plasmas testing negative for HBsAg can still transmit hepatitis B.

Probably, there is a relation between dosage and infectivity. As Tabor [16] has demonstrated, hepatitis B virus infectivity which might still be present in such plasmas or plasma derivatives may be neutralized by hepatitis B immunoglobulin. Therefore, addition of anti-HBs either during or after the manufacture of such products is a practical approach to prevent hepatitis B [17]. A similar immunologic neutralization of non-A/non-B hepatitis agent is not possible because neither the agent nor the protective antibody has been identified so far.

To reduce the risk of non-A/non-B hepatitis transmission, the manufacturer of fibrin sealant tests all donations of plasma for ALT levels. As early as 4 years ago serum alanine aminotransferase in donors could be shown to have a correlation with the risk of non-A/non-B hepatitis transmission [2, 3, 4]. However, experience has shown that rigorous quality control criteria – every donation with ALT levels ≥ 25 U/liter (25°C reaction temperature) is discarded and excluded from processing – reduce non-A/non-B hepatitis transmission, but do not eliminate it completely. The mechanism involved in the transmission of non-A/non-B hepatitis by fibrinogen or fibrin sealant was investigated in 1980 [18]. At that time, one lot of fibrinogen triggered non-A/non-B hepatitis in two patients and one patient developed chronically persisting hepatitis 2 years after the onset of the acute phase of the disease. The same lot of fibrinogen was injected intravenously into a chimpanzee in a concentration of 200 mg and produced typical non-A/non-B hepatitis with ultrastructural changes of the hepatocytes [19]. The chimpanzee developed an ALT level of 55 Karmen U/ml (five times the baseline 11 weeks after the intravenous administration of that fibrinogen lot). Two milliliters of pooled serum from samples drawn from that chimpanzee in weeks 4–10 postinoculation were given to another chimpanzee by the intravenous route. A typical non-A/non-B hepatitis developed in that chimpanzee 8 weeks postinoculation with that serum pool, manifesting itself in ALT increases of 4–5 times the baseline. In another study [20] a young chimpanzee was inoculated with ~100 mg of fibrinogen intravenously. The chimpanzee developed an ALT increase to 227 U/liter after a 16-week incubation period, with light microscopic and ultrastructural changes typical of non-A/non-B hepatitis. The two studies have shown that concentrations ranging from 100 to 200 mg may trigger non-A/non-B hepatitis if given intravenously. It must be borne in mind, however, that fibrinogen is not given intravenously when fibrin sealant is applied, but that clottable protein is transferred into a viscid solution which solidifies rapidly into a rubberlike mass after the addition of aprotinin, thrombin, and calcium chloride. The course of this solidification bears analogy with the physiological process of coagulation. For that reason, it is not likely that fibrinogen enters the circulation. It was the aim of this study to show that fibrinogen given in concentrations which produce non-A/non-B hepatitis if given intravenously, do not transmit non-A/non-B hepatitis if applied in the routine product combination.

Evaluation of the Risk of Hepatitis B Transmission

A prospective study on the viral transmission of hepatitis B carried out from 1979 to 1981 in the same department has shown 23 (or 0.52%) of 4400 pregnant women who were examined consecutively for the presence of hepatitis B markers to be antigen carriers [21]. The prevalence of HBsAg-positive pregnant women is determined by the ethnic composition of a patient population, particularly in countries with a low incidence of HBsAg (22). Sixty-five percent of the antigen carriers identified in the above study came from Southern Europe, Turkey, and the Philippines. The frequency of HBsAg carriers in the 3 year study varied widely. The small patient sample in the fibrin sealant study (68 evaluable patients out of 100) explains the nonrepresentative frequency of HBsAg and HBsAb in this group of women. Since in all samples (including the one taken preoperatively) HBsAb could be identified in only two patients, the percentage of patients considered to be immune to hepatitis B is too low, while the percentage of HBsAg carriers (2 of 68) is too high. One of the HBsAg carriers was a 29-year-old woman with an incompetence of the cervical canal who had a cerclage performed in the 17th week of gestation. HBs antigenemia in patients with normal liver function have been known for well over 4 years. The second case was a 33-year-old woman who had the same problem and the same intervention performed in the 15th week of gestation and gave birth in the 41st week. This patient had no history of HBs antigenemia and none of her relatives had hepatitis B.

The HBsAb which was detected in three patients on the 2nd and 7th postoperative days in concentrations of ≤ 15 mU/ml could not be clearly confirmed to have been HBsAb by inhibition. The concentrations were too low. HBcAb could not be detected. This suggests the HBsAb involved to probably have been a nonspecific one [23, 24].

In only one patient (group B) could HBsAb be detected 6 months after cerclage had been performed, in a concentration of 13 mU/ml. Since HBcAb was absent, this could not be considered a seroconversion. The results, therefore, suggest that fibrin sealant does not transmit hepatitis B, since none of the patients underwent hepatitis B infection serologically or clinically within the 6-month observation period.

Evaluation of the Risk of Non-A/Non-B Hepatitis Transmission

Since at the present time no serological test methods are available for the detection of non-A/non-B hepatitis virus(es) [25], the non-A/non-B hepatitis risk can only be assessed based on biochemical tests such as ALT or to a certain extent γ-GT. Some time ago determination of reverse transcriptase was described as an indicator of non-A/non-B hepatitis[26]. The sera available to us cannot be used for this determination, since this requires the plasma or serum samples to be deep-frozen at $-70°C$ immediately after they are taken, which was not done with the documentation samples collected. If typical clinical and biochemical findings were present, non-A/non-B hepatitis could only be diagnosed by exclusion of other forms of hepatitis, including cytomegaly and Epstein-Barr. Liver biopsies could not be taken for ethical reasons. Therefore, the risk of non-A/non-B hepatitis transmission was assessed based on elevated ALT and γ-GT levels. Numerous chimpanzee studies have shown that increases in ALT or γ-GT values beyond 2.5 times the baseline or normal upper limit are indicators of non-A/non-B hepatitis.

For well over a decade, statistically significant correlations have been known to exist among age, weight, sex, and enzyme activities. A correlation between weights and ALT levels is more markedly present in men than women. In women, on the other hand, age plays a more important role in younger women (below 30). The normal range of ALT values does not exceed 10 U/liter (0.95 quantile). In women between 30 and 40 years of age, the normal range lies between 5 and 21 U/liter with a median of 9 U/liter [9]. Studies on the normal range of ALT during pregnancy (where higher enzyme activities must in principle be expected) have not been done. The small patient sample did not allow stratification by age, body weight, or weeks of gestation if cerclage was involved. For all of the above reasons, the upper limit of the normal range was defined to be 20 U/liter and the limit beyond which non-A/non-B hepatitis was present was defined to be 50 U/liter (2.5 times the upper limit of normal). γ-GT levels were interpreted analogously. However, little is known about the correlation between γ-GT, age, weight, and sex.

Since γ-GT levels are also expected to be slightly higher during pregnancy, the upper limit of normal was again taken to be 20 U/liter and the limit for non-A/non-B hepatitis 50 U/liter (2.5 times the upper limit of normal). The slightly increased ALT levels of 41 and 46 U/liter 6 months postoperatively in the two patients in group B cannot be correlated with non-A/non-B hepatitis. In one patient ALT levels were increased 5 days before delivery of twins. In the other the increased enzyme activity showed 2.5 months postpartum.

The increased ALT levels of 46 and 40 U/liter in two patients, one in group A, one in group B, are below the defined limit for non-A/non-B hepatitis. The increased γ-GT value of 46 U/liter 10 weeks postoperatively in one patient (group A) cannot be interpreted as indicative of non-A/non-B hepatitis either.

Conclusions

Two-component fibrin sealant does not transmit hepatitis B or non-A/non-B hepatitis. Of 69 patients who qualified for evaluation of viral hepatitis transmission out of 100 entered into a randomized controlled study, none had hepatitis B, seroconversion, or clinically or biochemically manifest non-A/non-B hepatitis.

References

1. Seelich T, Redl H: Theoretische Grundlagen des Fibrinklebers. In: Fibrinogen, Fibrin und Fibrinkleber, ed. Schimpf K FK Schattauer Verlag, Stuttgart – New York, p. 199–208, 1980
2. Alter HJ, Purcell RH, Holland PV, Alling DW, Koziol DE: Donor transaminase and recipient hepatitis. Impact on blood transfusion services. Jama, 246:6, p. 630–634, 1981
3. Hornbrook MC, Dodd RY, Jacobs P, Friedman LI, Sherman KE: Reducing the incidence of non-A, non-B post-transfusion hepatitis by testing donor blood for alanine aminotransferase. N Engl. J Med, 307:21, 1315– 1321, 1982

4. Aach RD, Szmuness W, Mosley JW, Hollinger FB, Kahn RA, Stevens CE, Edwards VM, Werch J: Serum alanine aminotransferase of donors in relation to the risk of non-A, non-B hepatitis in recipients. N Engl J Med, 304:17, 989–1035, 1981
5. Empfehlungen der Deutschen Gesellschaft für Klinische Chemie. Z klin Chem u klin Biochem, 10, 182–192, 1972
6. Scheele J, Schricker K TH, Goy D, Lampe I, Panis R: Hepatitisrisiko der Fibrinklebung in der Allgemeinchirurgie. Med Welt, 32, 783–788, 1981
7. Panis R, Scheele J: Hepatitisrisiko bei der Fibrinklebung in der HNO-Chirurgie. Laryng Rhinol Otol, 60, 367–368, 1981
8. Synopsis der Leberkrankheiten. Editors: H Wallnöfer, E Schmidt und F W Schmidt. G Thieme Verlag, Stuttgart, 1974
9. Thefeld W, Hoffmeister H, Busch EW, Koller PU, Vollmar J: Referenzwerte für die Bestimmungen der Transaminasen GOT und GPT sowie der alkalischen Phosphatase im Serum mit optimierten Standardmethoden. Dtsch med Wschr, 99, 343–351, 1974
10. Persijn JP and W van der Slik: A new method for the determination of gamma-glutamyltransferase in serum. J Clin Chem Clin Biochem, 14:9, 421–427, 1976
11. Wüst H: Laboruntersuchungen. Klinische Gastroenterologie in zwei Bänden. Edited by L. Demling. Volume I: Diagnostische Übersicht, Mundhöhle und Rachen, Speiseröhre, Magen, Darm. 2. Auflage. G Thieme Verlag, Stuttgart – New York, 1984
12. Seagroatt V, Magrath DI, Ferguson M, Anderson SG, Schild GC, and CH Cameron: Preliminary evaluation of a collaborative study of the proposed British standard for hepatitis B surface antigen. Med Lab Sci, 38, p. 335–339, 1981
13. Barker LF, Gerety RJ, Lorenz DE, Rastogi SC and EB Seligmann Jr.: Biological standardization in viral hepatitis. In: Viral hepatitis. Eds. Vyas GN, Cohne SN, and Schmid R. The Franklin Institute Press, Philadelphia, 1978
14. Seeff LB: Hepatitis in hemophilia: a brief review. In: Frontiers in liver disease. Eds. Berk PD, Chalmers TC. Thieme Verlag Stratton Inc., New York, p. 231– 241, 1981
15. Hoofnagle JH: Hepatitis B surface antigen (HBsAg) and antibody (anti-HBs). In: Virus and the liver. Proceedings of the 28th Falk Symposium on the Occasion of the 5th Int. Congress of Liver Diseases 1979, p. 27–37. Eds. Bianchi L, Gerok W, Sickinger K, Stalder GA
16. Tabor E, Aronson DL, Gerety RJ: Removal of hepatitis B-virus infectivity from factor IX complex by hepatitis B immunglobulin. Lancet II, p. 68–70, 1980
17. Gerety RJ and Aronson DL: Plasma derivatives and viral hepatitis Transfusion 22:5, p. 347–351, 1982
18. Yoshizawa H, Akahane Y, Itoh Y, Iwakiri S, Kitajima K, Morita M, Tanaka A, Nojiri T, Shimizu M, Miyakawa Y, and M Mayumi: Viruslike particles in a plasma fraction (fibrinogen) and in the circulation of apparently healthy blood donors capable of inducing non-A/non-B hepatitis in humans and chimpanzees. Gastroenterology 79, 512–520, 1980
19. Jackson D, Tabor E, Gerety RJ: Acute non-A, non-B hepatitis: specific ultrastructural alterations in endoplasmic reticulum of infected hepatocytes. Lancet I, p. 1249–1250, 1979
20. Gudat F, Eder G, Eder C, Bianchi L, Stöcklin E, Krey G, Dürmüller U and HP Spichtin: Experimental non-A/non-B hepatitis in chimpanzees: light, electron and immune microscopical observations. Liver 3, p. 110–121, 1983
21. Sacher M, Eder G, Baumgarten K and H Thaler: Vertikale Hepatitis B Transmission. Ergebnisse einer prospektiven Studie 1978 bis 1981. Wr klin Wschr, 95–13, p. 447–451, 1983
22. Woo D, Cummins M, Davies PA, Harvey DR, Hurley R and AP Waterson: Vertical transmission of hepatitis B surface antigen in carrier mothers in two West London hospitals. Arch Dis Childhood 54, p. 670–675, 1979
23. Sherertz RJ, Spindel E and JH Hoofnagle: Antibody to hepatitis B surface antigen may not always indicate immunity to hepatitis B virus infection. N Engl. J Med, 309:24, 1983
24. Brotman B and AM Prince: Occurrence of AUSAB test positivity unrelated to prior exposure to hepatitis B virus. J Inf Dis 150:5, p. 714–720, 1984
25. Dienstag JL: Non-A, Non-B hepatitis. II. Experimental transmission, putative virus agents and markers, and prevention. Gastroenterology 85, p. 743–568, 1983
26. Seto B, Coleman WG jr, Iwarson S and RS Gerety: Detection of reverse transcriptase activity in association with the non-A/non-B hepatitis Agent(s). Lancet II, p. 941–943, 1984

II. Traumatology

Glueing of Osteochondral Fragments and Fixation of Dissecates in Osteochondrosis Dissecans

H. Zilch

Key words: Osteochondral fragments, osteochondrosis dissecans, fibrin sealant

Abstract

This is a report of our satisfactory experience in fixing 82 osteochondral fragments with fibrinogen glue, which we have used since 1979. This method has proven to be real progress in comparison with traditional fixation by screws or K-wires. The fragments were revascularized early. No second operation was necessary to explant metallic material. Fragments which were exposed to shearing forces were fixed in addition with splints of autogenous cortical bone, as we did in 25 cases. The joints must be immobilized for a period of 3 weeks.

In addition to the glueing of fragments we have used glue since 1978 to fix 22 vital dissecates in cases of osteochondrosis dissecans. First the bed must be prepared by reducing the sclerosis, by drilling the subchondral spaces and by transplantation of autogenous cancellous bone. Our experience with this method has also proved satisfactory.

Introduction

Since our experimental studies have shown that a narrow layer of fibrin can promote the appearance of capillaries in a bony transplant, while bigger clots of fibrin rather hinder quick revascularization during the first days [1], in 1979 we began with the glueing of fresh osteochondral fragments. Some time earlier we had already used fibrin glue for fixation of vital dissecates of osteochondrosis dissecans, after some preparation of the bed. Besides both these fields of application, of which the results are discussed in this paper, glue as a resorbable carrier for an antibiotic has proved satisfactory in treatment of osteitis in our clinic [2].

Glueing of Osteochondral Fragments

From 30 May 1979 until 31 December 1984 82 fragments were glued in 50 patients (average age: 21 years). Table 1 shows the distribution of individual fragments on various joints. There is a preference for the finger joints, the talus and the knee joint. The higher number of finger joints is based on the fact that our clinic is a center for replantation in Berlin and therefore a large number of patients with

Fibrin Sealant in Operative Medicine
Traumatology and Orthopaedics – Vol. 7
Edited by G. Schlag, H. Redl
© Springer-Verlag Berlin Heidelberg 1986

Table 1. Localization of the osteochondral fragments, (30. 5. 79–31. 12. 84)

	Patients (*N*)	Glued fragments (*N*)
Finger joints	10	22
Trochlea tali	16	21
Condylus femoris	9	15
Patella joint-surface	8	11
Caput radii (child)	4	8
Trochlea humeri	2	4
Malleolus medialis (joint surface)	1	1
	50	82

seriously injured hands are transferred to our clinic; on the other hand our main effort has been the glueing of the unstrained joint, to gather practical experience from this method.

Results

Three of the 82 glued fragments became detached during clinical treatment. Of these three patients, two had a fragment of the trochlea tali and one a fragment of the trochlea humeri. All three had not been immobilized postoperatively in the early phase of glueing. The detachments occurred during the 2nd week. In all three patients the fragments, even after fixation, were exposed to shearing forces because the bed was hardly excavated.

Apart from these primarily detached fragments no more loosenings were observed, and all patients had to undergo medical check ups to the time they were able to take up work; an additional 39 patients had follow-up examinations during a period of 8 months to 4.7 years (on average 2.1 years) after the operation. The results are summarized in Table 2.

Table 2. Results: osteochondral fragments

n 50 patients	(average age 23 years)
n 39 patients follow up	(average 8 months – 4.7 years) on average 2.1 years

Arthrotic alteration
    2 x finger joints
    1 x trochlea humeri
	3 patients

Minor complaints
    1 x finger joints
    1 x trochlea humeri
	2 patients

Limitation of joint movement
    2 x caput radii
    1 x trochlea humeri
	3 patients

Arthritic changes were found at three joints; two patients showed light discomfort and in three cases the movement was restricted. Glueing in the area of the trochlea humeri gave the poorest results since in one patient no healing was achieved and with the other patient arthritic changes as well as light discomfort and restriction in movement occurred. Because of the low case number concerning this joint general conclusions cannot be made.

Based on our practical experience we standardized the treatment of osteochondral fragments: When fragments cannot be protected from harmful shearing forces because of insufficient adaptation in a poorly excavated bed, additional possibilities of fixation must be chosen. In our cases the cornered splint of autogenous cortical bone proved successful, because the second operation for metal removal was not necessary. Despite this fact larger fragments had to be fixed with screws. All the glued osteochondral fragments were consequently immobilized in a cast splint for a period of 3 weeks and unburdened for 6–12 weeks, according to the localization.

Case Reports

The following are some examples of successful treatment and some cases with long-term follow-ups which were reexamined and accordingly testify to late results.

Case 1

Injury caused by a circular saw in a 25-year-old man, with destruction of the base of thumb joint after a subtotal amputation on 15 October 1979. The four osteochondral fragments were glued and both vessels and nerves were sutured microsurgically.

There was good mobility after 4.7 years and a sensitivity of 15 mm with two-point discrimination. X-ray showed good joint space and a small arthritic palmar osteophyte. For primary documentation 18 months after the injury, see [4].

Case 2

Thirteen-year-old girl with a fracture of the capitulum radii on 12 April 1980. The fragments were glued. One year after the accident the glueing zone still showed a cystic defect at the cancellous bone [4] that nowadays has largely refilled with new bone. After 4 years only a 10° reduction of pronation was left; the joint surface and space were satisfactory.

Case 3

Seventeen-year-old boy with a distorting injury of the right knee joint caused by a fall on 31 October 1980. Shearing of three osteochondral fragments at the lateral condylus of the femur. Refixation with fibrin glue. Symptom-free after 3.2 years. Wide joint space, no arthritic changes. For primary report 5 months after injury, see [3].

Case 4

Twenty-five-year-old man, whose trochlear tali split into four fragments after a fall 16 July 1982. The two larger fragments were fixed by screws while the smaller ones were attached by using fibrin glue. Two and a half years later he showed free mobility, pain-free stress and a radiologically satisfactory appearance. For a primary report 5 months after the injury, see [5].

Case 5 (Fig. 1)

Seventeen-year-old boy with a thumbnail-sized osteochondral fragment in the load-bearing area of the lateral condyle of the femur. Fixation with glue and angular splints of the cortical bone (9 May 1984). Ten months later the condition was normal.

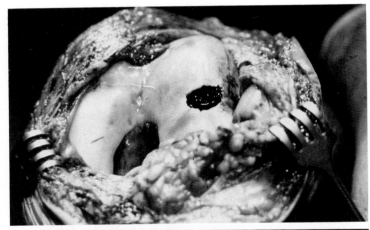

Fig. 1a

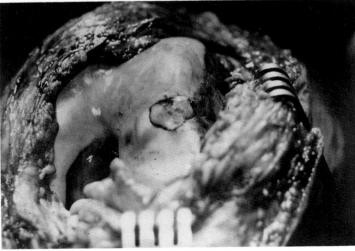

Fig. 1b

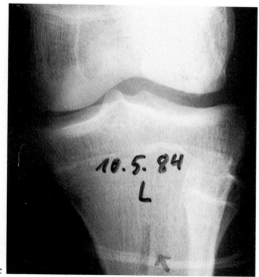

Fig. 1 c

Fig. 1 a–c. Case 5. *a* The bed of the osteochondral fragment at the medial condylus of the femur. *b* Refixation with fibrin sealant and angular splints of cortical bone. *c* The postoperative X-ray shows the area of the removed cortical splint *(arrow)*

Case 6 (Fig. 2)

Twenty-six-year-old man. Supination injury with rupture of the lateral ligaments of the ankle joint (21 February 1984) and a large lateral fragment of the talus dome. Twelve months later the condition was normal.

Osteochondrosis Dissecans

Osteochondrosis dissecans has proved to be an additional possibility while using fibrin glue, providing the separated portion contains the vital cartilage. The wide sclerosis especially in the bed must be milled out and drilled so that the cells out of the medullary space build up to a solid anchorage. As a rule, a bed treated in such a manner must be refilled with autogenous cancellous bone to keep the dissecat at the level of the joint surface. In the following cases concerning the condyle of the femur and the trochlea tali are given as examples.

Case 1 (Fig. 3)

A 24-year-old man with osteochondrosis dissecans of the condyle of the femur. Nearly free separated portion. The area of sclerosis was milled out, the autogenous cancelleous, bone was transplanted, and refixation with glue was carried out (July 1982).

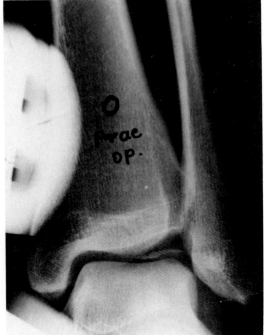

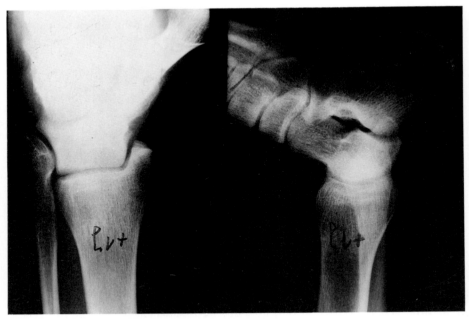

Fig. 2 a, b. Case 6. Osteochondral fragment of the talus dome before *a* and 1 year after *b* operation

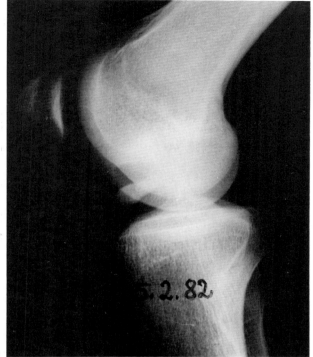

a

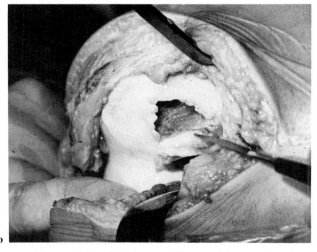

b

Fig. 3 a–f. Osteochondrosis dissecans of the condylus of the femur. *a* X-ray, *b* intraoperative view, *c* removal of the sclerosis area and filling of the subchondral space, *d* transplantation of autogenous cancelleous bone into the bed, *e* fixation with fibrin sealant *e* and *f* X-rays 2 years later

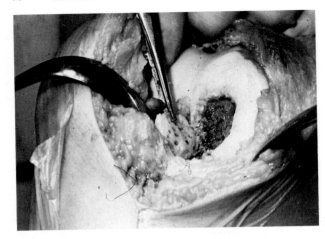

Fig. 3 c

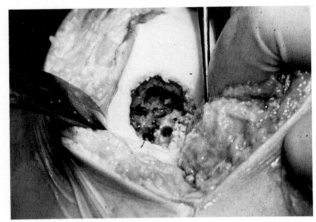

Fig. 3 d

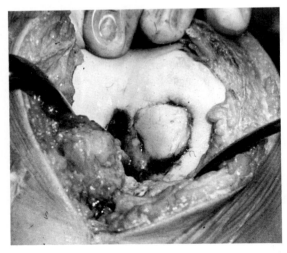

Fig. 3 e

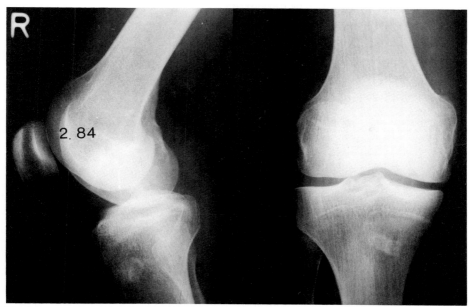

Fig. 3 f

Two years later, conditions were clinically and radiologically satisfactory. On arthroscopic examination the surface of the cartilage was found to be smooth and firm.

Case 2

A 19-year-old woman. Osteochondrosis dissecans on the medial dome of the talus. Same surgical procedure as shown in case 1. Two years later, smooth joint condition and symptom-free walking.

Number of Cases and Results

In addition to the glueing of fresh osteochondral fragments, we have refixed 22 separated portions since November 1978, with the above-mentioned method. Localization was the trochlea tali 12 times and the medial condylus of the femur in 10 cases.

One separated portion of the trochlea tali did not settle and had to be removed by a second operation. Fifteen patients, who underwent postoperative follow-up examinations during a period of 7 months to 3.7 years, showed radiologically satisfactory joint-surfaces and a free range of mobility concerning the upper ankle joint as well as the knee joint. However, after being put under heavy stress six of the patients experienced discomfort at some time, whereas two patients experienced very little. In six cases the talus and in two cases the condyle of the femur was concerned (Table 3).

Table 3. Results: osteochondrosis dissecans (*n*, 22 patients)

Healing	21
No healing	1 (trochlea tali)
Follow-up	7 months – 3.7 years postoperatively: 15 x
Radiologically O.K.	15 x
Minor complaints	6 x
Moderate complaints	2 x
Free movement	15 x

Discussion

Refixation of osteochondral fragments has succeeded due to the fact that it is only with this method that correct anatomical reconstruction is guaranteed. At first, possible use of fibrin sealant was given critical consideration since the glue lacks strong mechanical stability. But in animal experiments it was proven that in cases of small refixed fragments, after a period of 3 days, capillaries grew into the cancellous parts of the fragments [6]. This fact seemed to guarantee rapid healing.

Due to its poor mechanical firmness the glued fragments had to be sheltered from harmful shearing forces. This was accomplished by

1. Providing an excavated bed that fits exactly with the fragment
2. Additional fixation with angular splints of autogenous cortical bone, which were taken from the corticalis of the neighboring tube bone, obtained from the same incision
3. Immobilization of the joint for 3 weeks, independent of whether the method of glueing or additional cortical splints were used. For us 3 weeks seemed sufficient, because no loosenings of the fragment occurred after this period.

The question arises of whether due to the fragment size limitations exist in use of the glue. When applying the sealant, we only used fragments up to the size of 30 mm. Bigger fragments were screwed without additional glueing.

Follow-up examination by Paar et al. [7] showed that in the case of older fragments which had not been refixed in time, results were not as satisfying as in cases of immediate fixation. Our reported cases refer only to injuries that had been refixed within 1 day. It also has to be pointed out that the average age of our collective was 21 years and no patient was older than 30 years.

On the other hand good results were obtained in the case of osteochondrosis dissecans, as long as the separated portion seemed clinically vital and the bed had been thoroughly prepared.

References

1. Zilch H (1981) Der Einfluß des Fibrinklebers auf die Revaskularisierung des Knochentransplantates. Unfallheilkunde 83: 363–372

2. Zilch H, Drehsen R, Lambiris E, Hahn H (1982) Diffusionsverhalten von Cefotaxim aus der Fibrin-Antibiotika-Plombe im Tierversuch. In: Cotta H, Braun A (ed) Fibrinklebung in Orthopädie und Traumatologie. Springer Berlin Heidelberg New York pp 191–195
3. Zilch H, Friedebold G (1981) Klebung osteochondraler Fragmente mit dem Fibrinkleber – Klinische Erfahrungen. Akt Traumatologie 11: 136–140.
4. Zilch H, Friedebold G (1982) Klebung osteochondraler Fragmente und Fixierung von Dissecaten bei der Osteochondrosis dissecans. In: Cotta H, Braun A (ed) Fibrinklebung in Orthopädie und Traumatologie. Springer Berlin Heidelberg New York pp 142–145
5. Zilch H, Friedebold G (1983) Diagnostik und Therapie chondraler und osteochondraler Frakturen im Bereich des oberen Sprunggelenkes. Unfallheilkunde 86: 153–160
6. Zilch H (1980) Tierexperimentelle Untersuchungen zur Klebung kleiner osteochondraler Fragmente mit dem Fibrinkleber. Handchirurgie 12: 71–75
7. Paar O, Strubing W, Bernett P (1984) Die Knorpelklebung am Kniegelenk. Eine klinische Nachuntersuchung. Akt Traumatol 14: 15–19

Follow-up after Reattachment of Chondral and Osteochondral Fragments of the Knee Joint

T. Tiling

Key words: Arthroscopy, fibrin glueing, chondral fragment, osteochondral fracture, knee

Abstract

Chondral lesions must always be considered precursors of arthrosis. Chondral and osteochondral fragments of articulating joint surfaces must therefore be reconstructed. A precondition for this is a precise reattachment technique. Exact attachment of the detached pieces covering the whole lesion is made possible by fibrin glue. Implants should be avoided because they destroy the zone of regeneration – the chondral surface – and they necessitate a second operation. In this series of 21 cases, fragments were reattached, and 3 months after initial surgery, they were followed up arthroscopically. In 19 cases, good operative results were obtained.

Introduction

Chondral lesions of the hyaline cartilage are inevitable precursors of arthrosis since they can only heal in the sense of repairing the defect. Like no other diagnostic procedure athroscopy provides reliable information on the structure and extension of chondral lesions. Thus, we can recognize chondral evulsion fractures, which were formerly diagnosed during arthrotomy at an early stage. Therapy of acute bony or chondral lesions primarily involved the use of bone screws or Kirschner wire fixation. With this technique, only the larger osteochondral fragments were reattached. Chondral and small osteochondral fragments were not taken care of, and "defect healing" occurred through the eventual formation of fibrocartilage. Animal studies have shown that chondral and osteochondral fragments are incorporated into the lesion by natural healing and repair. This process does not take place in the repair margins of the fragment, where cartilage meets cartilage [1, 6]. Smaller fissures are closed with fibrocartilage coming from the floor of the fissure [2]. Good results have been reported based on clinical, radiographic, and occasional arthroscopic follow-ups [3, 4, 10].

Material and Methods

In 21 cases, chondral or osteochondral fragments resulting from an acute injury were refixed and documented from 1979 to 1983 at the University Hospital of Göttingen

Fibrin Sealant in Operative Medicine
Traumatology and Orthopaedics – Vol. 7
Edited by G. Schlag, H. Redl
© Springer-Verlag Berlin Heidelberg 1986

Table 1. Etiology of chondral and osteochondral fractures

Type of injury	n
Dislocation of the patella	12
Impact trauma	5
Distortion	3
Total	20

(Department of Surgery) and from 1984 onwards at the Surgical University Clinic, Cologne-Merheim, both in the Federal Republic of Germany. Acute trauma was defined as being an injury not older than 3 weeks. Chondral fragments were peeled off at the osteochondral border. Only fragments from the stressed areas or areas which could be stressed during a full range of motion of the knee were reattached. Dissected pieces which had been crushed were not treated. Furthermore, microsized crushed chondral and osteochondral fragments from nonstressed areas of the joint were extracted. The most common causes of injury (60%) were dislocation of the patella induced by impact trauma and distortion injuries (Table 1). Dislocation of the patella is always combined with avulsion injuries of the lateral condyle and less commonly with an additional fracture of the patella. Microscopically, the patella fragment shows multiple fissures and visible contusions around the fragment as a sign of chondral injury. The fragment of the lateral condyle usually presents no contusion fracture, since it is literally cut off [8]. Replantations were undertaken in 12 cases at the lateral condyle, in six cases at the patella, and in three cases at the medial condyle. In all, 13 osteochondral and eight chondral fractures were noted. The patella and lateral condyle proved to have twice as many osteochondral and chondral fractures as the medial condyle (Table 2).

The first ten refixations were performed without fibrin glueing. The crushed chondral margins were not smoothed. In the following 11 cases, chondral and osteochondral dissections were smoothed, and the overlapping laminar cartilage was cut off. Loosened cartilage around the defect was glued back into its original position, as was the dissected piece itself. Additionally, a screw fixation was used in

Table 2. Location and type of injury in 21 chondral and osteochondral lesions

Location		n
Patella (n = 6)	chondral	2
	osteochondral	4
Medial condyle (n = 3)	chondral	2
	osteochondral	1
Lateral condyle (n = 12)	chondral	4
	osteochondral	8
Total		21

two cases and Kirschner wire fixation in one case. Patients treated by means of internal fixation received primary functional treatment postoperatively. In contrast, patients treated by fibrin glueing were immobilized for 3 weeks with secondary functional treatment. Increasing weight bearing was started at 9 weeks postoperatively. In three cases, the result was verified through arthrotomy to remove screws from the patella. Otherwise, arthroscopy was used. The Kirschner wires were removed extra-articularily.

Of 20 patients, 18 were absolutely free of symptoms during the 2-year follow-up period. Three months after the first operation, two patients showed complete chondral destruction of the patella fragment. This was discovered by follow-up arthroscopy. Both patients belonged to the first series of cases which did not receive fibrin glueing. The destroyed parts had to be smoothed. Subsequently, patients complained of pain and, clinically, presented chondropathy of the patella. For 19 lesions, we were able to demonstrate good results at follow-up. In cases where the chondral surface was not primarily damaged, it was seen to be smooth and could not be depressed with the instrument. The area that had once been fragments had the same color as the area around the original injury. At the border of the replanted chondral or osteochondral fragment, either craterlike defects or fissures filled with fibrocartilage could be seen. The inlet screws or Kirschner wires were overgrown by chondral tissue. Where Kirschner wires had been used, visible iron deposits partly punctuated and partly enlarged by areas of yellowish-black or brownish discoloration were noted.

However, there were fundamental differences in the results of the two groups. The group being treated with fibrin glue always showed fibrocartilage that had filled out the defects, whereas in the group without fibrin glueing, craterlike defects were noted. The operative performance of one patient was so poor that we had to reoperate 3 weeks after the acute trauma. In this case, there was extensive destruction of the medial condyle with five osteochondral fragments. The injured and bruised area was filled with connective tissue without any sign of bony healing of the refixed fragments. The connective tissue was removed and the matrix of the defect filled with spongy bone. The condyle was then reconstructed with the fragments glued into place and additionally fixed with Kirschner wires. At follow-up arthroscopy, all the fragments had healed, but of course the damaged surface remained. Two years postoperatively, the patient was free of symptoms with a free range of motion and no effusion into the knee joint.

Those fragments which had been attached only with fibrin glue did not show increased softening of the chondral surface (as a consequence of immobilization) compared with those patients treated without fibrin glue. Significantly, biopsies from the replanted fragment and the area surrounding the injury did not show significant catabolism of the matrix when either chondral or osteochondral fragments were damaged. The chondral cells were intact. Dotted islands with increased cell turn-over (showing cell compensation for cartilage catabolism) were not noted [9].

Discussion

Chondral and osteochondral injuries of the knee are the most common conse-
quences of a patellar dislocation. Since clinical signs are easily overlooked, it is
absolutely mandatory to examine by means of arthroscopy every knee which has
suffered from acute trauma and shows blood effusion. Otherwise, the extent of
chondral lesions cannot be properly recognized. Of 90 dislocations of the patella,
there was refixing of fragments in 12 cases. Our experience has shown that not only
osteochondral, but also chondral lesions should be reattached since they heal
perfectly into the defect, leaving only a small, clinically unimportant fissure.
Replantation is possible if the chondral and osteochondral fragments are big enough
and not too bruised. Furthermore, they should be in areas of the joint where
cartilage surfaces are stressed or two cartilage surfaces articulate against each other.
Smaller fragments should be removed arthroscopically. Arthrotomy is not advisable
because it would mean more trauma to the joint that would outweigh the benefit
derived from reattaching tiny fragments. In areas with high stress which bear
chondral lesions, one should also consider replacing the chondral fragments by
osteochondral transplantation. The question is whether this leads to better postoperative results. Apart from this, acceptable results and symptom-free normal
function can be achieved if operative techniques are good and all minor fractured
chondral fragments are removed. Lifted chondral areas should be refixed with fibrin
glue. Cartilage has proved to develop an internal tension which leads to elevation of
the edges if the fragment is centrally fixed by screws or Kirschner wires. As a
consequence, nutrition – which comes through the bone below the fragment – is
jeopardized. If fibrin glue is used, there is sufficient adhesion between the fragment
and the underlying bone. It is important that only an extremely thin layer of glue be
applied between the bone and the fragment. Pressure should be applied for at least 5
min. The reabsorption of the fibrin leads to bone healing and thus guarantees the
survival of the hyaline cartilage. In adults, injuries and lesions of cartilage surfaces
are irreversible. That is why one should refrain from reattachment with splints,
screws, or wires. Our arthroscopic follow-up examinations showed that, in every
case where only fibrin glue was used, it was possible to achieve a secure attachment.
One exception has to be made, and this is when chondral fragments are located on
convex joint surfaces. These should be secured by Kirschner wires which have to be
fixed extra-articularly to avoid a situation where the tension of the cartilage lifts the
chondral fragments because the adhesive strength of the glue is insufficient. Another
definite advantage of using fibrin glue is the fact that only one operation is
necessary. The advantages of fibrin glueing are listed below:

1. Exact positioning of the small osteochondral fragments
2. Only means of attaching chondral fragments successfully
3. No additional iatrogenic trauma
4. Improved adaptation of fissure
5. Sealing of the fracture fissure
6. Improved revascularization allowing removal implants

If the chondral wound is sealed off with fibrin glue from the synovial fluid,
chondral edema and catabolism of the matrix are reduced. This may explain why

there are no crater-like lesions around the fragments in cases where fibrin glue is used, whereas multiple similiar defects were seen in cases where fibrin glue was not applied.

References

1. Braun A, Brüwer W, Schumacher G, Heine WD (1979) Die fibrinolytische Aktivität im traumatisierten Kniegelenk und ihre Bedeutung bei der Fibrinklebung osteochondraler Frakturen. Hefte Unfallheilkunde 138: 814
2. Cotta AH, Puhl W (1976) Pathophysiologie des Knorpelschadens. Hefte Unfallheilkunde 127: 1
3. Gaudernak T, Skorpik G (1983) Klinische Erfahrungen mit dem Fibrinkleber bei der Versorgung von osteochondralen Frakturen. Hefte Unfallheilkunde 163: 317
4 Glückert K (1985) Arthroskopische Kontrolluntersuchungen nach Klebung osteochondraler Frakturen am Kniegelenk. In: Scheele J (ed) Fibrinklebung, Springer. Berlin Heidelberg New York Tokyo p 198
5. Paar O, Bernett P, Erhard W (1985) Versorgung chondraler und osteochondraler Frakturen am Knie und oberen Sprunggelenk mit Fibrinkleber. In: Scheele J (ed) Fibrinklebung, Springer. Berlin Heidelberg New York Tokyo p 193
6. Passl R, Plenk H jr, Sauer G, Spängler HP, Radaszkiewicz T, Holle J. Die homologe reine Gelenkknorpeltransplantation im Tierexperiment. Arch Orthop Unfall Chir 86: 243
7. Puhl W, Dustmann HO, Quosdorf U (1973) Tierexperimentelle Untersuchungen zur Regeneration des Gelenkknorpels. Arch Orthop Unfall Chir 74: 362
8. Röddecker K, Fricke D, Tiling Th (1985) Patellaluxation und Knorpeltrauma. In: Hofer H (ed) Fortschritte in der Arthroskopie. Enke Stuttgart p 74
9. Tiling Th, Schmid A, Fricke D (1985) Arthroskopische Kontrolle nach Refixation chondraler und osteochondraler Fragmente. In: Hofer H (ed) Fortschritte in der Arthroskopie. Enke Stuttgart p 47
10. Zilch H, Friedebold G (1981) Klebung osteochondraler Fragmente mit dem Fibrinkleber, klinische Erfahrungen. Akt Traumatol 11: 136

Applications of Fibrin Sealing in Sports Traumatology

O. Paar and P. Bernett

Key words: Osteochondral fracture, ligamentous rupture, therapy, fibrin glueing

Abstract

The application of fibrin adhesive in operative medicine and surgery has led to a broader field of indications. In the beginning this adhesive was only used in the reconstruction of cartilage or bone-cartilage fragments, but now it is increasingly being applied for the reconstruction and repair of ligaments and tendons, especially the Achilles tendon. The following paper is a report on our experience in this respect.

In 1909, Bergel reported about the utilization of fibrin in human medicine. However, the method of fibrin sealing was first described during World War II by Michael and Abbott as well as by Cronkite in the fields of skin transplantations, nerve sealing, and hemostasis. Experimental works by Matras et al. in 1972 were the basis for its practical application in traumatology and orthopedics for the sealing of traumatized structures.

The principle of fibrin sealing is the reconstruction of the final phase of blood clotting; a highly concentrated fibrinogen solution is brought to coagulation with a thrombin solution.

With increasing clinical experience the indications for fibrin sealing changed. Initially used for cartilage surgery, fibrin sealant is now used successfully for the reconstruction of tendons and ligaments. In sports traumatology we find the following indications:
1. Reconstruction of joint surfaces by replantation of detached cartilage, or rather cartilage–bone fragments
2. Adaptation of Achilles tendon ruptures
3. Reconstruction of fibular ligaments of the ankle joint
4. Fine adaptation after transcondylar suture at the cruciate ligament in the knee
5. Reconstruction of the inner ligament in the knee

Chondral and Osteochondral Lesions

In joints under extreme stress, such as the ankle and the knee, cartilaginous lesions are especially critical. They constitute the etiopathogenetic factor for the development of a joint arthrosis and lead to a change in the joint mechanics and subsequently to a reduction of the stress-bearing capacity of the joint. In order to reconstruct the joint surface and thus the physiological stress-bearing capacity of the cartilage and to minimize unfavorable effects of chondrosynovial retroactions on the total cartilage, it is necessary to reconstruct the joint as fast and exactly as possible.

Before the introduction of fibrin sealant in surgical therapy, recent osteochondral chips were refixed by bone bolting, screwing, or Kirschner's wire. However, only larger osteochondral fragments could thus be replaced while smaller parts or chondral fragments alone could not be refixed due to lack of fixation possibilities. The only alternative was spongylization of the ulcus basis to promote growth of granulation tissue.

Fibrin sealant has enlarged the spectrum of therapies in chondral surgery. Even smaller defects can now be sealed with hyaline cartilage. Thus a gap in the list of treatments could be fined.

The advantages of fibrin sealing are:
1. Sealing of smaller or several small fragments
2. Sealing of chondral fragments (Figs. 1, 2)
3. Simple sealing technique
4. No rearthrotomy for metal extraction
5. No additional lesions by metal parts of chondral fragments or adjacent joint surfaces

Our Own Experience

Since 1978 67 chondral and osteochondral fractures in the knee and the ankle have been sealed. In the knee, we had 38 cases of recent traumata; five cases were older chondral defects (6–14 days) with degenerative changes of the remaining cartilage and 5 cases were even older traumata (>14 days) with onset of degeneration also of the adjacent cartilage. In 21 cases findings could be arthroscopically evaluated, at an average of 19 months after surgery. In 17 patients chondral findings were uneventful. The reimplanted fragment had grown in, and the adjacent cartilage showed no degeneration. In four cases the implanted fragment was destroyed, and in two of these cases even dislocated.

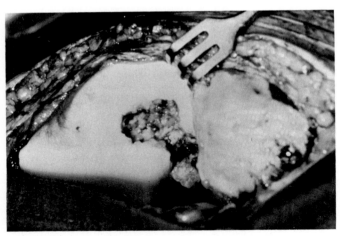

Fig. 1. Osteochondral fracture in the stress-bearing zone of the medial femoral condyle in the knee

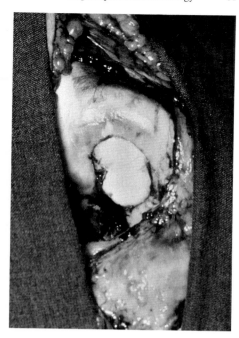

Fig. 2. After reimplantation with fibrin sealant the chondral fragment is evenly fitted in the defect

In the talus, 19 chondral fragments were reimplanted with fibrin sealant. In the majority of cases, the cartilage had detached from the lateral talus edge due to a supination trauma. The cases are continously ambulantly followed up, whereby the surgical results are evaluated both clinically and radiographically. Up to this day we have not had any signs of progressing chondral degeneration or of dislocation of the fragment. The majority of patients reengaged in sports.

Achilles Tendon

Clinical experience has shown that Achilles tendon sutures lead to complications in about 5% of cases. These are very small necroses which tend toward fistula formation and reruptures. Even pathological changes of the tendon attachment at the calcaneus are occasionally observed in the postoperative phase; they are probably a consequence of a rupture healed in shortening.

Two considerations are decisive for the utilization of fibrin sealant. As far as sports are concerned, the majority of our patients are strongly motivated and need a fully functioning muscle–tendon apparatus in order to be able to fulfill all sporting demands. On the other hand, the tendon stumps are often considerably traumatized, so that adaptation sutures could not be fastened in elongated, thinned, and split tendon tissue. The tendon fasciae can be much better united with fibrin sealant.

Intraoperatively it is necessary to split exactly the proximal and distal tendon stumps so that the rupture sites, present in several layers, can be clearly exposed. By combing the tendon stumps, the rolled up fasciae and those already adhering to each other are stretched and smoothened. Then the individual fasciae are reconstructed step by step with fibrin sealant and finally the peritendineum is closed with adsorbable single-knot sutures. A central supporting suture secures the two tendon stumps and increases the stability of the reconstructed tendon.

Our Own Experience

Since 1983 we have reconstructed 21 Achilles tendons with fibrin sealant (18 recent injuries, < 2 days; 3 older injuries, > 3 days). Patients were immobilized for 6 weeks, and subsequently treated with therapeutic exercises, so that they could take up their sporting activities after about 6 months. Up to now, we have had no reruptures or achillodynia (Figs. 3, 4).

None of the patients showed excessive stress-specific swelling tendency of the para-achillean soft tissue after removal of the plaster. We found no adhesions and the motility of the tendon was not reduced. Computer tomography carried out about 7 months after surgery revealed nearly physiological density; the values, averaging 98 HU (Hounsfield Units), were almost in the standard range.

The Fibular Capsula–Ligament Apparatus in the Upper Ankle

Many clinical observations have shown that the surgical reconstruction of the fibular ligament apparatus is much more successful than conservative therapy. The aim of

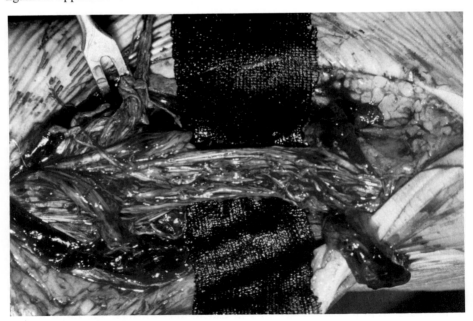

Fig. 3. Achilles tendon rupture at the typical site

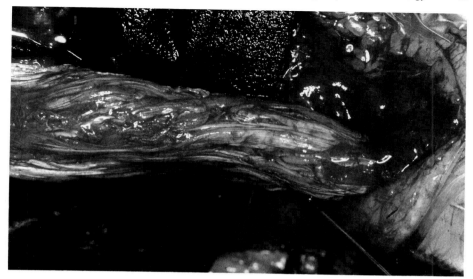

Fig. 4. Restoration of the continuity of the tendon with fibrin sealant

the surgical intervention is to create the prerequisites for healing with as little granulation tissue as possible or for the formation of a stable granulatory surface. Ligament stumps should be joined exactly and as atraumatically as possible so that the full stress-bearing capacity of the ligament apparatus is restored and scar insufficiencies are avoided. Thus, more pre-existing ligament tissue is preserved and scarring at the suture sites is considerably reduced.

However, there are cases in which the ligament stumps are damaged so severely that they can only be insufficiently reconstructed with adaptation or transosseous sutures. In addition, 5%–8% of surgeries have shown scar insufficiencies which have led to luxation of the ankle.

Especially in medial or distal ruptures the calcaneofibular ligament is especially affected by healing disturbancies, which lead to distinct scarry changes. Very often we find the fasciae split and elongated and the stumps thinned so the application of adaptation sutures is almost impossible. In addition, sutures lead to very small necroses, which in their turn bring about tissue reactions.

In these cases fibrin sealant is a real alternative to sutures. Sealing, according to our experience, has the following advantages:
1. Successful reconstruction without vast exposure of soft parts
2. No tendon necroses due to adaptation sutures
3. The previous length of the tendon is almost always achieved
4. Anatomical reconstruction
5. Atraumatic procedure
6. Shorter duration of surgery

Our Own Experience

Since 1984, we have reconstructed nine calcaneofibular ligaments with fibrin sealant. For better exposure of the operation site we used Hohmann's levers which push the fibular tendon sheath sufficiently aside to obtain a better view of the distal tendon insertion.

Postoperative treatment does not differ from those cases treated with adaptation sutures.

Anterior Cruciate Ligament

In recent lesions of the anterior cruciate ligament we try to preserve preexisting tissue and to restore the continuity of the cruciate ligament. In proximal, or rather medial ruptures, we apply plaited sutures and the ligament is attached by transosseous fixation. In 57 cases we used fibrin sealant for fine adaptation of the individual fasciae, so that the rupture sites are intimately closed. In addition, we reinforced the sutured and sealed ligaments with the distally stemmed semitendinosus tendon, which was previously synthetically reinforced. This combination graft is led by the "over the top" technique to the lateral femoral shaft and fixed there with screws.

Inner Ligament of the Knee

In recent lesions of the soft parts of the knee we often find severe traumata not only of the anterior cruciate ligament but also of the inner ligament. Especially in cases of distal ruptures of the inner ligament, the ligament stumps often show considerable disintegration. Splitted and elongated stumps are difficult to reconstruct since adaptation sutures cannot be secured and tend to rupture. Fibrin sealant allows restoration of the continuity of the ligament in the original length and in its anatomical course. In some individual cases reinforcing grafts consisting of autologous, or rather allogeneic materials are necessary for better securing of the reconstruction result.

Discussion

The introduction of fibrin sealant in surgical medicine has considerably enlarged the spectrum of treatments in sports traumatology. Used in the beginning mainly in indications of chondral traumatology, the sealant is now increasingly used in surgery of tendons and ligaments. Fibrin sealant helps in the management of traumatized structures by simplifying the surgical techniques, by making atraumatic surgery possible, by shortening the duration of the surgical intervention, and by reducing the complication rate.

References

1. Bergel S (1909) Über Wirkungen des Fibrins. Dtsch Med Wochenschr 35:663
2. Cronkite EP, Lozner EL, Deaver JM (1944a) Use of thrombin and fibrinogen in skin grafting. JAMA 124:976
3. Gebert L, Hene R (1983) Subcutane Achillessehnenruptur. Nachuntersuchungsergebnisse zur standardisierten Nahttechnik. Unfallheilk 86:525
4. Glückert K, Pesch HJ, Czerwenka R (1980) Ergebnisse der Sehnenklebung im Experiment und in der Klinik. H Unfallheilk 148:818
5. Matras H, Dinges HP, Lassmann H, Mammoli B (1972) Zur nahtlosen interfascikulären Nerventransplantation im Tierexperiment. Wiener Med Wochenschr 122:517
6. Michael G, Abbott W (1943) The use of human fibrinogen in reconstructive surgery. JAMA 123:279
7. Paar O, Strübig W, Sernett P (1984) Die Knorpelklebung am Kniegelenk, eine klinische Nachuntersuchung. Akt Traumatol 1:15
8. Paar O, Bernett P (1984) Therapie der Achillessehnen-Ruptur beim Sportler. Vorteile der Fibrinklebung. Fortschr der Med 43:46
9. Wrus U, Vecsei V, Hetz H, Czerwenka R (1980) Ergebnisse der Sehnenklebung im Experiment und in der Klinik. H Unfallheilk 148:818

Biomechanical Properties in Osteochondral Fractures Fixed with Fibrin Sealant or Kirschner Wire

J. Keller, T. T. Andreassen, F. Joyce, V. E. Knudsen, P. H. Jørgensen, and U. Lucht

Key words: Fibrinogen, fracture fixation, biomechanics

Abstract

The aim of the study was to evaluate the development of mechanical strength and adaption of the fragments after fibrin sealing of an osteochondral fracture. In mongrel dogs, a standardized osteochondral fracture was performed in both the medial and lateral condyle of the left femur and fixed with fibrin sealant or Kirschner wire. After glueing a plastic cylinder to the fragment, mechanical testing of the fragment was possible. The model was convenient for comparing different fixation techniques, as the contact area of the fragments was of equal size in both the fibrin and Kirschner wire group. Adaption of the fragments and mechanical strength were compared after 4, 7 or 8 and 14 days after operation. The initial mechanical strength in osteochondral fractures fixed with fibrin sealant was low, but the development of mechanical strength seems to be rapid in the first 2 weeks of healing. The adaption of the fragments was better in the fibrin sealed group than in the Kirschner wire group. Fibrin sealant can be used for the fixation of small osteochondral fractures, when sufficient immobilization is achieved.

The present study was undertaken to evaluate the development of mechanical strength and the displacement of the fragments in a standardized osteochondral fracture fixed with fibrin sealant or Kirschner wire.

Materials and Methods

Adult mongrel dogs were used. Under sterile conditions, a lateral arthrotomy of the left knee was performed. The patella was dislocated medially, the tendon to the extensor digitorum longus muscle divided, and the infrapatellar corpus adiposum resected. The knee was then flexed maximally and an osteochondral fracture was made to a depth of 3–4 mm in the distal articulating surface of both the medial and lateral condyle of the femur with a specially designed circumferential saw mounted on a standard drill (Fig. 1). The cartilage anterior to the 7-mm-diameter cylinder was resected. Then, the cylinder was resected just under the bone/cartilage interface with a 6-mm-osteotome at a depth of 1.5 mm and at an angle of 30° (Fig. 2). After removal, the smallest and largest heights of the fragment were recorded. The fragments were fitted into the condylar defects.

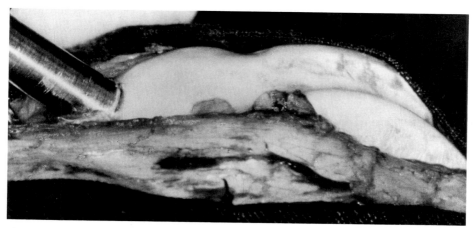

Fig. 1. Performance of the standardized osteochondral fractures with a special circumferential saw

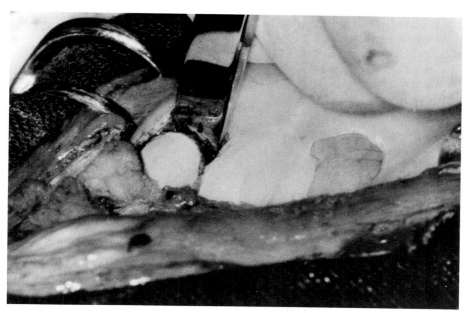

Fig. 2. The osteochondral fragment is cut off with an osteotome

After random allocation, one fragment was fixed with Kirschner wires and the other with fibrin sealant. Two 1.0-mm-Kirschner wires were drilled through the medial and lateral aspects of the condyles. The wires were inserted so deeply that they did not protrude above the surface of the cartilage and the opposite ends were bent and buried in the periosteum. Approximately 0.1 ml dog fibrin seal ($\sim$ 80 mg/ ml clottable protein) and 0.1 ml of a solution containing thrombin (250 IU/ml), aprotinin (3000 IU/ml) and CaCl (20 mM) was mixed and applied to the other defect in the femur. The corresponding fragment was placed in the defect and gentle pressure applied for 5 min. The knee was fully extended and the leg immobilized in a brace taped to the foot.

The dogs were killed 4, 7, 8 and 14 days after operation and the displacement of the fragments was evaluated and rated on a semiquantitative 1–4 scale (1, elevation more than 0.5 mm in $> 180°C$ of the fragment circumference; 2, $< 180°$ and $> 90°C$; 3, $< 90°C$ and $> 0°C$, 4, no elevation at all).

For mechanical testing, the distal femur was mounted in a specially designed cage allowing traction force perpendicular to the fracture line by glueing a 5-mm plastic cylinder to the fragments with cyanoacrylate (Fig. 3). The setup was mounted in a materials-testing machine (Alvetron 250, Lorentzen and Wettre) and traction applied with a constant speed of 10 mm/min while load and deformation were recorded. The area between the load-deformation curve and the deformation-axis to the point where failure becomes evident represents the energy absorption of the fracture.

The study of the initial strength of the fibrin sealant in osteochondral fractures performed as described previously was carried out in the right leg of the dogs killed. The measurements were performed 1/2 h after application of the sealant using the same procedure as described above.

For statistical significance, the mechanical results were analyzed by a t-test after assuring homogeneity of variances and normal distribution. The semiquantitative data were analyzed by Fisher's exact test. The results are expressed as the mean ± SEM.

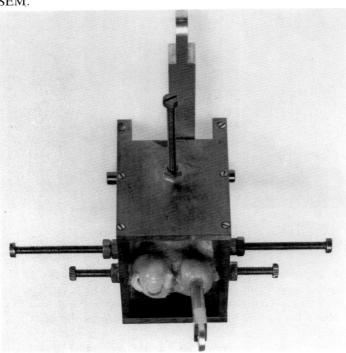

Fig. 3. Distal femur mounted in the cage and the plastic cylinder glued to the medial fragment

Results

The contact area of the fragments in the fibrin sealant group was 0.67 ± 0.02 cm^2 and 0.66 ± 0.01 cm^2 in the Kirschner wire group. The contact area of the fragments in the in vitro investigation was 0.65 ± 0.02 cm^2.

In the fibrin sealant group, significantly fewer fragments were displaced compared with the Kirschner wire group (Table 1). Figure 4 shows two fragments with no elevation at all after 14 days of healing. None of the knees were macroscopically inflamed. In the Kirschner wire group, the underlying semilunar cartilage was damaged in one case.

The maximum tensile strength in the fibrin sealed fragments was initially 0.7 ± 0.1 N/cm^2 and the failure energy 0.04 ± 0.01 N/cm^2.

Table 1. The displacement of the fragments after healing

	Fibrin sealant (N = 19)	Kirschner wire (N = 19)
No elevation at all	18	12
Elevation more than 0.5 mm in < 90°	1	1
Elevation more than 90° > and < 180°	0	6
Elevation more than > 180°	0	0

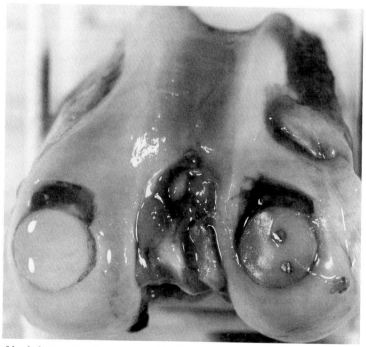

Fig. 4. Ideal healing of both fragments after 14 days of healing

After 4 days of healing in the fibrin group the maximum tensile strength was 5.1 ± 0.8 N/cm^2 and the failure energy 0.25 ± 0.04 N/cm^2. In the Kirschner wire group after 4 days of healing the maximum tensile strength was significantly decreased (2.6 ± 0.1 N/cm^2) compared with the fibrin group but no significant change in failure energy was found (0.20 ± 0.03 N/cm^2). After 7 or 8 days of healing, 8 knees were tested. Two fragments fixed with fibrin sealant and four fixed with Kirschner wire separated through the fracture line, while the other separated through the cyano-acrylate bond. When adding setter to the glue, breakage of the cyanoacrylate bond occurred between 35 and 63 N/cm^2. After 14 days, no fragments could be separated in the fracture line.

Discussion

The contact area of the fragments was almost the same in the fibrin sealant group, the Kirschner wire group and in the in vitro study. Thus, the model is appropriate for comparing different fixation techniques.

The fragments were not exactly congruent to the fracture site of the femor condyle. This might be the reason that the initial maximum tensile strength in this study was much smaller than reported by Claes et al. [2]. In their model, the surfaces were planed with a microtome before sealing.

The small fragments could easily be replaced at the femoral fracture site using fibrin sealant. During the drilling of the Kirschner wires through the fragments, it was difficult to keep them in exact position and this might explain the poorer adaptation after healing in the Kirschner wire group.

The initial mechanical strength of the fibrin sealed fragments was very low, but after 4 days of healing the strength increased sevenfold and after 14 days the fragments had a maximum tensile strength of more than 35 N/cm^2. To prevent dislocation, reliable immobilization is necessary for the first weeks of healing. This is in accordance with the observations of Braun et al. [1], who reported that fibrin fixated osteochondral fractures often fall off when no immobilization is used.

We find that the model is convenient for comparing different fixation techniques. The initial mechanical strength in osteochondral fractures fixed with fibrin sealant was low, but development of mechnical strength seems to be rapid in the first 2 weeks of healing. The adaption of the fragment was better in the fibrin sealed group than in the Kirschner wire group. Fibrin sealant can be used for fixation of small osteochondral fractures, when sufficient immobilization is achieved.

References

1. Braun A, Schumacher G, Heine WD (1982) Fibrin-Klebung osteochondraler Fragmente im Tierexperiment. In: Cotta H, Braun A (ed) Fibrinkleber in Orthopädie und Traumatologie. 4. Heidelberger Orthopädie-Symposium. Georg Thieme Verlag Stuttgart, New York, p 110
2. Claes L, Burri C, Helbing G, Lehner E (1982) Die Festigkeit von Knorpelklebungen in vitro. In: Cotta H, Braun A (ed) Fibrinkleber in Orthopädie und Traumatologie. 4. Heidelberger Orthopädie-Symposium. Georg Thieme Verlag Stuttgart, New York, p 106

Clinical Experiences Using Fibrin Sealant in the Treatment of Osteochondral Fractures

T. Gaudernak, B. Zifko, and G. Skorpik

Key words: Fibrin sealant, osteochondral fractures

Abstract

Since 1977 we have used a fibrin sealing system for the replantation of osteochondral fragments. In more than 100 cases of osteochondral replantation which have been followed up at regular intervals, the use of this sealant has been found clearly superior to other methods. Due to the excellent adhesive strength no additional osteosynthesis is usually necessary. The eventual operative result depends on the condition of the cartilage surface and to a considerable degree also on the optimal management of concomitant damage to ligaments.

Flake fractures are most frequently seen in displacement of the patella and subluxation of the talus. In both types of injury replantation of the flakes with fibrin sealant promises good results. Furthermore, the sealing technique is an apt tool in the hands of an experienced surgeon for the management of lesions to the cap of the head of femur and comminuted joint fractures. The fact that longer immobilization may be necessary in some cases is compensated for by the good results to be attained by this method.

Introduction

Osteochondral Fracture

The direct or indirect impact of force on cartilage leads to flake fracture in, or rather on, the subchondral layer or to separation of the cartilage portion together with the underlying bone, possibly even with the spongiosa (osteochondral fracture in the strict sense of the word). In comminuted joint fractures, avascular bone fragments, torn off together with cartilage portions, are frequently seen; these, as well as the above-mentioned osteochondral fragments, can be readily reimplanted.

Osteochondrosis Dissecans

Whereas in osteochondral fractures the blood supply of the osseous bed is good — usually bleeding from fresh bone wounds is quite severe — the situation is entirely different in osteochondrosis dissecans. Both in the separated portion and especially

Fibrin Sealant in Operative Medicine
Traumatology and Orthopaedics – Vol. 7
Edited by G. Schlag, H. Redl
© Springer-Verlag Berlin Heidelberg 1986

in the so-called osseous bed circulation is disturbed. In addition, degenerative changes are present, and this is why we prefer the term osteochondrosis. There are good chances of healing, provided the osseous bed and the portion to be replanted are treated appropriately.

Fibrin Sealing System

Since 1977 we have used a fibrin sealant (Immuno AG) for the reimplantation of osteochondral fragments. The essential advantage of this sealant in comparison with other products is its excellent tissue compatibility along with sufficient adhesive strength. Thus, additional methods of osteosynthesis are rarely required. We have used lyophilized fibrin sealant ever since it became available. A double syringe application system is easy to handle and allows precise and deft application of the sealant, especially when the high thrombin concentration is used.

Sealing Technique in Fresh Osteochondral Fractures

The condition of the osseous bed is of decisive importance: it must be free from clotted blood and fresh bleeding. If there is any uncertainty as to the vascularization of the bone, drilling and curetting may be required to uncover sufficently vascularized bone for early union of the fragment to the vascular system.

The cases we have operated on so far have been limited to the gluing of osteochondral fragments. When the cartilage portion was very small, the subchondral bone underneath the cartilage to be replanted had to be drilled several times to ensure bone healing. When followed up radiologically, partial calcification of the basal cartilage layers is visible later on.

If the fragment fits perfectly into the recipient bed, application of a few drops of fibrin sealant and compression for 3 min (use watch for control) are sufficient to attain stability (Fig. 1). Difficulties arise when the cartilage is enlarged due to edema, or the bone fragment to be replanted is severely damaged by contusion, laceration or fracture and thus cannot be easily replaced into its bed. In these cases the recipient bed should be trimmed. In superficial chondral fractures it may also be necessary to trim the cartilage. Depressions should be packed with a mixture of fibrin sealant and cancellous bone.

However, in our experience, cartilage trimming requires great caution. It seems preferable to seal even multiple cartilage fractures with fibrin sealant (Fig. 2).

Postoperative immobilization in a plaster cast usually varies between 3 and 6 weeks. Limited weight-bearing of the cartilage is desirable, except for extensive

Fig. 1. Ideal conditions for the replantation of an osteochondral fragment. The cartilage of the flake to be replanted is largely intact and has been torn off together with the adjacent portion of subchondral bone. The cancellous bone of the osseous bed is still bleeding. In this case the fragment can be easily fixed with fibrin sealant; additional osteosynthesis is not necessary. It is essential to correct subluxation of the patella laterally by plication of the medial, and release of the lateral, retinacula

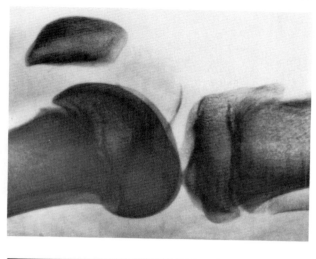

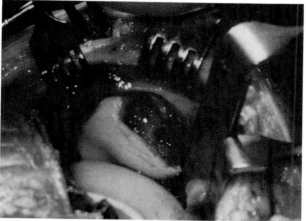

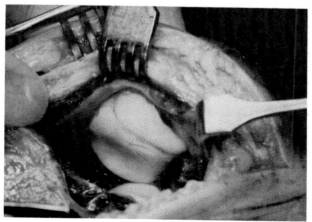

Fig. 1

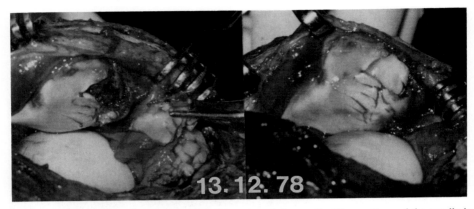

Fig. 2. Sixteen-year-old male patient with dislocation of the patella. The cartilage of the patella is severely comminuted medially; one larger fragment has also been torn off. After fixing the fragment with fibrin sealant and smoothing the cartilage, the longitudinal cartilage fractures are likewise filled with the sealant. Following surgical correction of the retinacula, the limb is immobilized in plaster for 4 weeks. Four years and 6 months later, slight calcification of the basal cartilage layers in the area of the medial surface of the patella is evident radiologically. Clinically, the patient is without symptoms. He is pursuing sport again

comminuted joint fractures where weight-bearing may not be allowed for a period of 16 weeks or more. In these cases it is useful to apply a splint, brace, or similar apparatus to prevent weight-bearing.

Applications and Results of Sealing Osteochondral Fragments

Since 1977 we have performed more than 100 osteochondral replantations. Most of our cases are documented photographically and have been followed up radiologically and clinically once a year.

Osteochondral Fractures in the Area of the Knee

Chondral flake fractures of the *medial surface of the patella* are the most frequent injuries caused by dislocation of the patella, which often passes unnoticed. Since we started to perform routine arthroscopy of every hemarthrosis of uncertain origin, osteochondral fracture of the knee has become a far more common diagnosis (Fig. 1–4).

Within 1 week of injury the conditions for restoration are still ideal in most cases. But we also had a patient in whom successful replantation was performed even 17 days after injury and the result finally attained was excellent.

As a rule, the fragments are quite large; the osseous portion should be at least half the size of the cartilage area. Owing to the traumatic mechanism leading to dislocation of the patella, cartilage damage and fractures, which may essentially

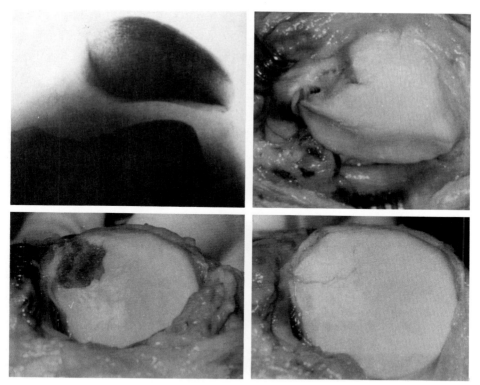

Fig. 3. Thirty-four-year-old male patient with slipping patella. Radiologically, there is no evidence of a flake fracture. Arthrotomy reveals considerable cartilage depression and a chipped bone fragment, which can be readily reduced. In this case, too, subluxation of the patella has to be corrected

compromise the result, are frequent. If optimal reduction of the fragment is prevented by chondral edema, it is of advantage not to trim the cartilage, but to restore its original shape by compression osteosynthesis (Fig. 4). It is essential to correct subluxation of the patella or a slipping patella by reinforcement of the retinacula, if necessary also by transference of the tibial tuberosity. Depending on the concomitant injuries, the limb is encased in plaster for 4 in 6 weeks.

Osteochondral Fragments of the Lateral Condyle of Femur

Usually, this type of lesion is likewise caused by displacement of the patella. Often the osteochondral fragments are still attached by the synovial membrane and, in that case, can be readily replanted. Again it is necessary to correct the slipping patella by plication of the medial and release of the lateral retinacula, if necessary even by transference of the tibial tuberosity.

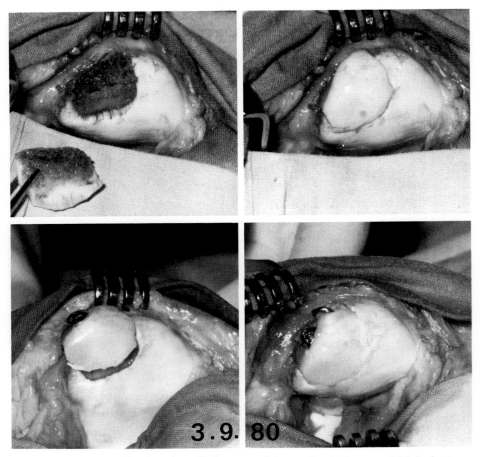

Fig. 4. Eighteen-year-old male patient; displacement of the patella with large medial flake fracture, which lends itself to replantation. As cartilage swelling prevents ideal reduction of the fragment (*top, right side*) compression osteosynthesis by screw is applied and the fibrin sealant injected before tightening the screw. In this case, the advantage of the sealant is tight closure of the cartilage lesion and precise tissue union

Osteochondral Fractures of the Medial Condyle of Femur

Such lesions are rare, but can be repaired with fibrin sealant in the same manner.

Results

In all 29 patients with osteochondral fractures in the area of the knee, whose injuries date back more than 2 years and who have been followed up at regular intervals, bone healing has been achieved, while in 3 patients flexion is restricted by 10°;

movement is entirely unimpaired in the rest. Twenty-two patients have no symptoms what so ever, and seven have slight complaints such as sensitivity to weather changes and problems when climbing stairs.

The clinical result of replantation is essentially dependent on the concomitant cartilage defect.

Replantation of Osteochondral Fragments of the Lateral Ridge of Talus

Flake fractures of the lateral ridge of talus are frequent and are often concomitant lesions of subluxatio tali supinatoria. The fragments torn off are mostly 10 x 10 to 10 x 20 mm in size and, unless comminuted, can be satisfactorily replanted. The torn ligaments are sutured, and the lower leg has to be immobilized in plaster for 6 weeks postoperatively. Weight-bearing is allowed after 4–5 weeks, depending on the location of the fractured flake.

Thirteen patients, injured more than 2 years previously, have been regularly followed up. In eight cases ideal operative reduction has been achieved; in five cases the postoperative X-rays still show a narrow line between the fragment and its osseous bed. No healing of the fragments has been attained in two patients, who have, however, absolutely no complaints. In six patients healing has been ideal; in two cases the replanted fragment is slightly depressed: one fragment is tilted. One patient developed osteochondrosis dissecans, as evident from the X-ray. In one case reoperation was necessary, as displacement of the replanted fragment was seen on X-ray during routine postoperative re-examination. This was a case from the beginnings of the method, when we had little experience with the sealing technique.

Seven patients are without signs of arthrosis; five patients developed slight, and one patient moderate arthosis.

Eight patients have regained full range of motion of the ankle joint; in five patients motion is slightly restricted (up to 10°). Nine out of 13 patients are fully capable of practising sports again (Fig. 5).

Flake Fractures of the Medial Ridge of Talus

These are considerably less frequent in our patients and mainly occur in combination with other severe lesions of the ankle joint. In these cases replantation is also possible.

Further Applications of the Replantation of Osteochondral Fragments

Osteochondral flakes torn off from the head of femur as a result of dislocation of the hip are usually readily fixed with fibrin sealant. Even in three cases of extensive, comminuted fracture of the head of femur, where osteosynthesis by screws was performed to join major fragments, small osteochondral flakes in between were fixed with fibrin sealant. In five other cases, fragments in the weight-bearing area have been replanted.

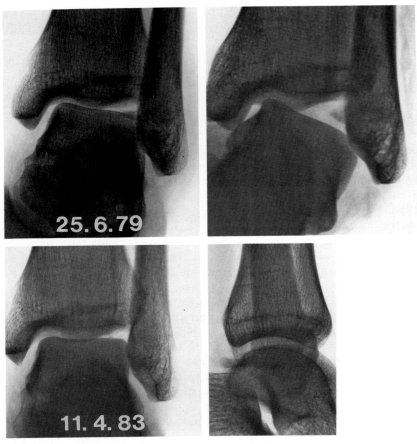

Fig. 5. Typical subchondral flake fracture on the lateral edge of talus caused subluxation of the talus. After replanting the fragment with fibrin sealant and correction of the lateral ligaments of the ankle joint the lower leg was immobilized in plaster for 6 weeks. The case has been followed up for a period of 4 years: the clinical and radiological results are excellent

The results are encouraging, but the observation periods are too short to permit final conclusions (Fig. 6). In osteochondral fractures of other articulations, such as the interphalangeal joints, the head of radius and the head of humerus, the fibrin sealant can also be used for the replantation of fragments. When interphalangeal joints were affected, our results were not as good, but these were usually open fractures.

Fig. 6. Thirty-four-year-old male patient with flake fracture in the weight-bearing area of the cap of the head of femur as a result of hip displacement in a skiing accident. After conservative management the fragment was lodged in the intraarticular space so that open surgical reduction was necessary. The fragment was fixed with fibrin sealant; as, in addition, extensive cartilage damage had been caused, Voss' myotenotomy was performed. Healing has been without complications. The

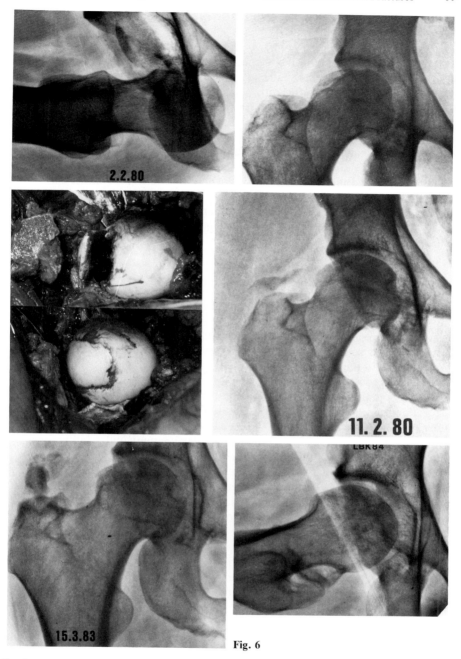

Fig. 6

patient has no symptoms and practises sport again. Clinically, abduction is limited by 15°; otherwise motion is unimpaired. Three years after injury the X-ray still shows an area of increased opacity of the cancellous bone underneath the replanted fragment; the outline of the head of femur is slightly irregular, but smooth; the articular space is not narrowed. The patient is scheduled for reexamination

Sealing Technique in Osteochondrosis Dissecans

Both in the knee and in the ankle we prefer to perform arthrotomy and extirpation of the focus with access from the chondral side. The necrotic portion is carefully removed and several holes made in it with the air drill. Then the bony bed is carefully trimmed until sufficiently vascularized bone has been uncovered. The resulting cavity is packed with a mixture of fibrin sealant and autologous spongiosa, and the necrotic portion, interspersed with spongiosa, is fixed with the sealant (Fig. 7).

By this surgical technique and subsequent immobilization in a brace to prevent weight bearing, radiologically evident bone healing and freedom from complaints has been achieved in three cases of osteochondrosis dissecans of the talus. In five patients with osteochondrosis of the medial condyle of femur, the limb has been immobilized in plaster for 6 weeks postoperatively and weight bearing limited to 20 kg. Clinically, all five patients have no symptoms; in one patient the focus can be still recognized on X-ray.

Discussion

Several treatment modalities of osteochondral fractures and of osteochondrosis dissecans are described in the literature. Obviously, there is no concurrence on this subject matter, the only agreement being that the treatment of osteochondrosis dissecans is problematical.

In our opinion it is of fundamental importance to discriminate between osteochondral fracture, being a fresh lesion, and osteochondrosis dissecans, which is a degenerative process.

In our opinion, prompt replantation of the fragment and fixation with fibrin sealant is superior to all other techniques.

The conservative treatment recommended by some authors seems to be highly questionable, primarily because of the uncertainty of the diagnosis. Since we started to perform an arthroscopy of every hemarthrosis in the knee of uncertain cause, we know of the discrepancy between the often harmless X-ray findings and the real damage.

If the osteochondral fragment is removed, fibrocartilage tissue grows into the defect. This chondral scar tissue is inferior to hyaline cartilage and thus inadequate in weight-bearing areas. But when these fragments are replanted, especially juveniles and young adults stand a good chance of full restitution which should not be missed.

As compared with other methods, one of the advantages of the sealant is its easy application (e.g., the seamless fixation of a fragment with cortical nails is far more difficult). But also fixation by wiring is usually not as satisfactory as with fibrin sealant. Osteosynthesis by screws transfixing the articular cartilage not only causes additional cartilage damage, but also necessitates a second intervention.

The fact that in some cases longer immobilization is necessary is not a serious drawback, as usually concomitant lesions of ligaments by themselves require longer

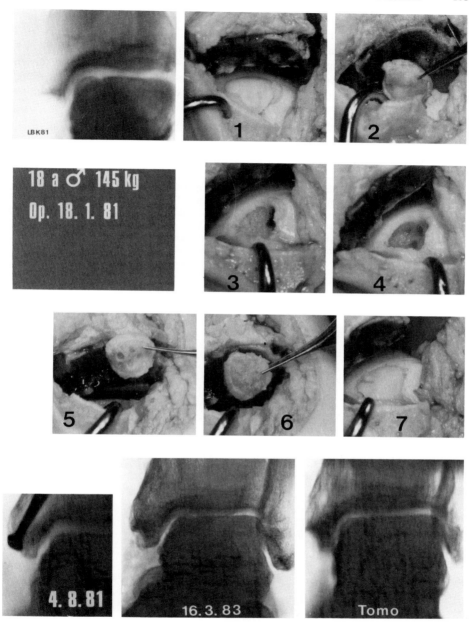

Fig. 7. The technique of operative management in osteochondrosis dissecans on the medial edge of talus: by osteotomy and reflection of the inner ankle, the necrotic portion is uncovered and cautiously lifted from its bed with a fine spatula. On *pictures 2 and 3* the sclerotic bone of the removed portion and of the osseous bed can be clearly seen. On *pictures 4 and 5* the osseous bed and the fragment have been trimmed prior to the introduction of a mixture of spongiosa and fibrin sealant and replantation of the fragment. After 7 months complete healing has been attained. At the last annual check the X-ray was still excellent; the patient is without symptoms

periods of fixation. Thus, there is no need for the osteosynthesis to reach a degree of stability tolerating joint movement.

If it is expected, or cannot be prevented, that the glued fragment is subject to shearing forces, or in extensive comminuted joint fractures, additional osteosynthesis with wire or screws is indicated. In these cases the sealant is used to protect the cartilage lesion from the synovia and to promote vascularization of the replanted fragments.

References

1. Gaudernak T (1982) Klinische Erfahrungen mit dem Fibrinkleber bei der Versorgung von Knorpel-Knochenfragmenten und Dissekaten. In: Fibrinkleber in Orthopädie und Traumatologie (Cotta H, Braun A), Georg Thieme Verlag, Stuttgart, New York, 158–167 (mit ausführlicher Literaturübersicht)
2. Zilch H, Friedebold G (1983) Diagnostik und Therapie chondraler und osteochondraler Frakturen im Bereich des oberen Sprunggelenkes. Unfallheilkunde, 86, 153–160

Histological Observations After Replantation of Articular Cartilage Using Fibrin Sealant

R. Passl and H. Plenk Jr.

Key words: Articular cartilage replantation, fibrin sealant, histomorphology

Abstract

Based on encouraging results with the fixation of pure articular cartilage with fibrin sealant (FS) in animal experiments, pure cartilage (and osteochondral fragments) were replanted in human patients using FS.

From individual cases, biopsies could be taken from macroscopically not well healed areas during arthroscopic examination. The histological results from these cases are presented, together with the overall clinical experience.

Six weeks after operation, the graft showed no union with the subchondral bone and was separated from the cartilage bed in the area examined. However, after 3 months, the grafted cartilage fused with the subchondral bone, but pannus-like tissue covered the surface and the cleft at the border to the bed. After 1 and 5 years, complete fusion with the subchondral bone and the surrounding cartilage can be demonstrated. There is only covering pannus at the latter observation time. In the majority of the 43 cases treated so far, excellent results were obtained, enabling the patients to take up their sporting activities again.

Introduction

In contrast to bone tissue, articular cartilage shows only insufficient capacity for repair [1]. Therefore, while osteochondral fragments can be refixed using various procedures [7] and will heal in the subchondral bone layer, pure cartilage fragments will be mostly removed and, e.g., drill holes are made in the subchondral bone in order to facilitate the ingrowth of reparative granulation tissue. Since in our experience the traumatic avulsion of pure cartilage occurs as frequently as that of osteochondral fragments [4], the results of our animal experiments on the transplantation and replantation of pure cartilage using different adhesives [2, 5] led to the clinical application of fibrin sealant [6] for the replantation of not only osteochondral but also pure cartilage fragments. The clinical results obtained so far will be presented here, together with the histomorphological evidence of the fate of these grafts as observed in biopsies taken during arthroscopic examination.

Fibrin Sealant in Operative Medicine
Traumatology and Orthopaedics – Vol. 7
Edited by G. Schlag, H. Redl
© Springer-Verlag Berlin Heidelberg 1986

Material and Methods

Since 1974, when a large cartilage fragment was successfully replanted to the medial femoral condyle of a 13-year-old football player [3], we started in 1980 routinely to replant large cartilage fragments by using fibrin sealant (Tissucol, Immuno AG, Vienna) when they were detected during arthroscopy of a traumatic hemarthrosis, and so far altogether 43 cases have been treated by this procedure (Table 1). Cartilage fragments were considered large when their diameter was greater than 1 cm in the knee joint and greater than 0.5 cm on the tarsus. For the fibrin sealant, the original technique [6] was used with slight modifications (see manufacturers instructions, Immuno AG, Vienna). In individual cases, when there were old cartilage fragments lacking adaptability to the curvature of the defect, the replants were additionally secured by Kirschner wires.

Table 1. Localization of the 43 cartilage fragments replanted with the fibrin sealant from 1980 to 1985

Location	Number of cases
Patella	12
Lateral femoral condyle	9
Medial femoral condyle	15
Trochlea of the talus	7

In most of the cases only clinical follow-up controls were possible, but in about one-third an arthroscopic examination could also be performed. In five of these latter cases (Table 2) a cartilage-bone biopsy could be taken from the border of the replant in an area which looked altered or not well healed arthroscopically. The instrument was a core trephine, with an inner diameter of 2 or 4 mm. The biopsies were fixed in Schaffer's fixative (neutral formalin: 80% ethanol = 1:3), embedded in methylmethacrylate, and undecalcified microtome sections were stained with different staining procedures (see figure legends).

Table 2. Histories of the five cases examined arthroscopically and histologically in this study

Case No.	Age (years)	Initial trauma	Time after operation	Reason for examination
1	20	Traffic accident	6 weeks	Journey abroad
2	16	Kick in the knee	3 months	Recurrent hemarthrosis
3	18	Traffic accident	3 months	Metal removal
4	16	Kick in the knee	1 year	Renewed trauma
5	23	Concrete slab against the knee	5 years	Renewed trauma

Results

The results obtained clinically can be classified as excellent. Most of the (young, sporting) patients, after 1 year of restricted activities, could take up their normal athletic activities again. So far, only in 2 cases out of the 43 treated by this procedure was a failure observed: In a young male patient with an old osteochondrosis dissecans, the fragment became loose and had to be screwed on again. In a 45-year-old male with a defect of the anterior cruciate ligament the replant was glued into a cartilage ulcer. Despite an unusually long plaster cast fixation (6 weeks) the replant loosened and had to be removed during arthroscopic examination.

Arthroscopic and Histological Observations

Six weeks after the operation, the cartilage replant is found in place, but looks whiter and feels softer than the surrounding cartilage. However, there is a distinct cleft at the border of the replant where the curvature of the condylar roll comes to the edge. The biopsy taken from this area shows that the replant is not united with the subchondral bone and with the cartilage bed (Fig.1). In the cleft, granulation tissue which is partly transformed into fibrocartilage is found, and remnants of apparently the fibrin sealant can be seen between the trabeculae of subchondral bone.

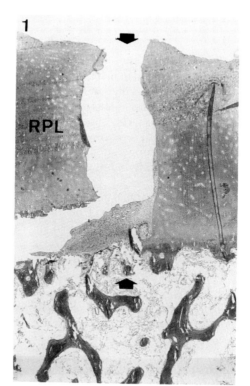

Fig. 1. Marginal biopsy of a cartilage replant, 6 weeks after operation. The cartilage replant *(RPL)* is separated from the bed by a wide cleft *(arrows)* which contains granulation tissue at the bottom. (Trichrome-Goldner stain, × 80).

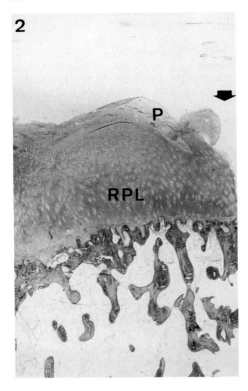

Fig. 2. Marginal biopsy of a cartilage replant, 3 months after operation. The cartilage replant *(RPL)* is firmly united with the subchondral bone, but separated from the surrounding cartilage by a cleft *(arrow)* and covered with pannus *(P)*. (Toluidine blue stain, × 80).

Three months after the operation, arthroscopy reveals in both cases that the replants are healed in nicely and display a firm consistency. Their borders, however, are easily recognizable, and the somewhat sunken-in surface is covered by pannus tissue. The biopsies taken from these areas show an irregular surface (Fig. 2) with the covering pannus. The subchondral bone, however, has united with the replant without visible difference to the surrounding cartilage bed.

One year after operation, the cause for the recurrence of hemarthrosis after a new trauma could be found in a detached small osteochondral fragment from the tip of the patella. The large replant on the lateral condyle, however, has almost completely healed in. Only at the border of the normally looking and consistent replant a small pannus is projecting from the surface (Fig. 3). The biopsy taken from this area shows the border between replant and cartilage bed now totally fused and filled with a perpendicularly oriented fibrocartilaginous tissue which projects over the surface (Fig. 4). No difference is found in the subchondral bone layer.

Five years after the operation, a fresh ligament strain after an old meniscus injury caused much more damage to the condyle adjacent to the worn down meniscus, while the replant looked virtually intact. The biopsy was taken from the replant border and showed a perfectly normal subchondral bone layer, but a distinct step at the transition to the surrounding cartilage (Fig. 5). The surface of the replant is uneven and covered with organized (fibrocartilaginous) pannus. Except in the cartilage structure, the union of the replanted cartilage with the bed is no longer visible.

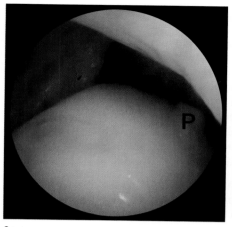

3 a

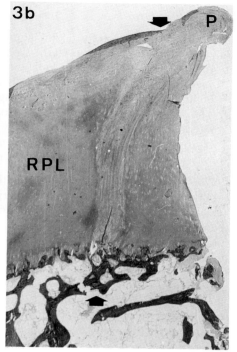

Fig. 3 a u. b. Arthroscopic view *(a)* and marginal biopsy *(b* Trichrome-Goldner stain, × 80) of a cartilage replant, 1 year after operation. Only a small, rod-like pannus *(P)* is projecting at the former cleft *(arrow)* between the cartilage replant *(RPL)* and bed. Note the uniform subchondral bone layer!

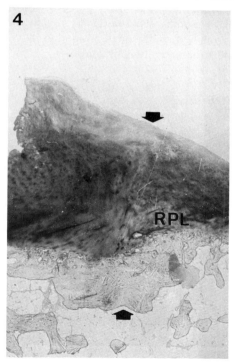

Fig. 4. Marginal biopsy of a cartilage replant, 5 years after the operation. Only by its cellular architecture the uneven surface of the articular cartilage allows estimation of the position of the former cleft *(arrows)*, but there is a distinct step in the subchondral bone layer. (Giemsa stain, × 80).

Discussion

The ethical justification for taking biopsies after apparently successful replantation of cartilage fragments in this study is given for the following reasons:

1. In all of our cases there was great interest on the part of the patients themselves (and their parents) in establishing that the cartilage replant had fused with the bone, in order to plan further sporting activities or to obstain from them.
2. The biopsies were always taken from areas which arthroscopically showed alterations, and never from apparently intact or not damaged areas. Thus, taking the biopsy can be considered as not more harmful than the shaving procedure with subsequent Pridie-drilling which is routinely performed in such cases.

The histological observations made in this material greatly resemble the histological findings reported in our animal experiments [2, 5]. Our histomorphological and clinical experiences with this procedure so far can have considerable significance for the therapeutic strategy of such injuries, since cartilage which is detached from subchondral bone in the mineralization zone shows normally no greater tendency for reunion. A cartilage ulcer with no load bearing capacity at all will result and persist for years, and post-traumatic arthrosis is unavoidable. After the usual procedure of removing the cartilage fragment and drilling holes into the subchondral bone layer, a fibrocartilaginous repair tissue can fill in the defect, but mostly in an insufficient way. With larger defects a loadable joint will be never restored. On the contrary, replantation of large cartilage fragments using the fibrin sealant has resulted in most of the cases treated so far in painless, loadable joints which looked excellent from a clinical and arthroscopic point of view, and this healing seems to be achieved after 6–12 months. Therefore, the replantation of also pure cartilage fragments can be strongly recommended as an alternative to the procedures currently in use for this posttraumatic joint situation.

References

1. Otte P (1972) Die Biologie des Gelenkknorpels im Hinblick auf die Transplantation. Z Orthop 110: 677-695
2. Passl R, Plenk H Jr, Sauer G, Spängler HP Jr, Radaszkiewicz T, Holle J (1976) Die homologe reine Gelenksknorpeltransplantation im Tierexperiment. Arch orthop Unfall-Chir 86: 243-256
3. Passl R, Plenk H Jr, Sauer G, Egkher E (1979) Fibrinklebung von Knorpelflächen. Experimentelle und klinische Ergebnisse. Med u Sport 19: 23-28
4. Passl R, Schopp E (1985) Diagnostik und Therapie frischer Knorpelläsionen. In: Hofer H (ed) Fortschritte der Arthroskopie. Enke, Stuttgart, p 44.
5. Plenk H Jr, Passl R (1980) Trans- and replantation of articular cartilage using the fibrinogen adhesive system. In: Gastpar H (ed) Biology of the Articular Cartilage in Health and Disease. Schattauer Stuttgart-New York p 439.
6. Spängler HP Jr. Holle J Braun F (1973) Gewebeklebung mit Fibrin. Wien klin Wschr 85: 827–831
7. Zilch M, Friedebold G (1981) Klebung osteochrondaler Fragmente mit dem Fibrinkleber. Akt. Traumatol 11: 136-148

Reconstruction of Post-traumatic Bone Defects with a Spongiosa-Fibrin Glue-Plug

B. STÜBINGER, R. KETTERL, and R. LANGE

Key words: Fibrin glue, spongiosa transplant, post-traumatic bone defect

Abstract

The reconstruction of post-traumatic bone defects by spongiosa transplantation remains a challenge to therapy in traumatology. Based on our previous experimental studies, we used a mixture of spongiosa with fibrin glue in 102 patients with bone defects caused by trauma or by radical surgical debridement in cases of post-traumatic osteitis. In 95% of the patients, only one operation was needed to achieve functionally sufficient reconstruction with the spongiosa fibrin glue plug. Postoperative follow-up examinations showed that signs of acute infection subsided by the second and fourth postoperative week. Increased scintigraphic activity was found in the spongiosa-receiving area for the first 4 months postoperatively. Thereafter, X-rays showed complete ossification and the scintigraphic activity returned to normal. Based on these results, we recommend the use of the spongiosa fibrin glue plug for post-traumatic bone reconstruction as opposed to spongiosa alone.

Introduction

Filling of large bone defect cavities and bridging of long shaft discontinuities, such as result from either trauma itself or from debridement in cases of post-traumatic osteitis, remain a therapeutic challenge in clinical traumatology. The osteoblastic transformation of spongiosa, which is transferred into such defects, depends primarily on the early proliferation of new blood vessels from the surrounding tissue into the transplant.

Studies on dog tibias from our institution showed that the addition of fibrin glue to the transplanted spongiosa results in its earlier vascularisation, when compared with the use of spongiosa alone [5]. Similar results have been reported by others (1/6/7). Based on these studies we have been using the combined spongiosa-fibrin-glue-plug for bridging of bone defects at the Chirurgische Klinik und Poliklinik of the TU Munich for the last 5 years.

Fibrin Sealant in Operative Medicine
Traumatology and Orthopaedics – Vol. 7
Edited by G. Schlag, H. Redl
© Springer-Verlag Berlin Heidelberg 1986

Table 1. Localisation and number of the treated bone defects

	n
Lower leg	67
Thigh	14
Forearm	16
Upper arm	5
	102

Methods

From January 1979 until August 1985 we used the spongiosa-fibrin-glue-plug in 102 patients. Eighty-two of these patients received spongiosa for filling of bone defects, which had resulted from radical debridement in cases of post-traumatic osteitis. The remaining 20 patients suffered from large trauma-induced defects and had no previous history of infection. The total group studied consisted primarily of males (the ratio of males to females being 4:1) and the average age of the whole group was 37.4 years (17–69 years).

The frequency and localisation of the treated bone defects are shown in Table 1.

Operative Procedure

The first step in the operative preparation of the spongiosa-receiving bed should be radical debridement of avascular and necrotic tissue. In cases of post-traumatic osteitis, it is our policy to wait until the acute signs of infection have subsided before we transplant the spongiosa in a second step operation.

Following removal of the autologous spongiosa (only if absolutely necessary do we combine autologous with homologous spongiosa, at a ratio of 1:1), fibrin-glue (Tissucol) is added in a ratio of fibrin-glue to spongiosa of 1:20. This mixture, which we call the spongiosa-fibrin-glue-plug, is then fitted tightly into the defect. In a last step we coat the spongiosa by an additional thin layer of fibrin-glue, in order to ensure a firm connection between the transplant and the surrounding areas and fibrous tissue.

All patients undergo periodic postoperative examinations (including clinical observation, determination of WBC (white blood cells) and ESR (erythrocyte sedimentation rate), X-rays and scintigraphy) until ossification of the spongiosa is completed.

Results

In 95% of the patients (i. e. 96 out of 102), complete reconstruction of bone defects was achieved by just one, primarily autologous or autologous/homologous spongiosa-transplant with fibrin-glue. In five patients a second transplant was needed.

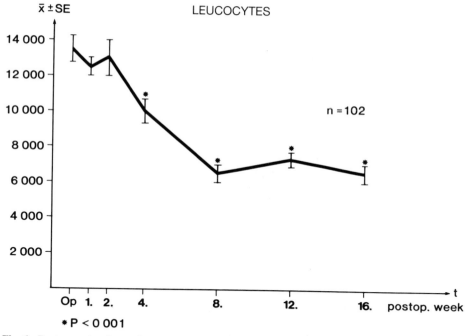

Fig. 1. Postoperative determination of WBC in patients treated with spongiosa-fibrin-glue-plug

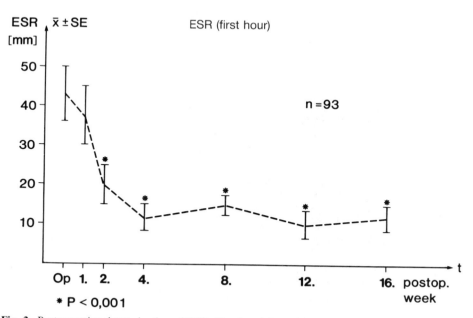

Fig. 2. Postoperative determination of ESR (first hour) in patients treated with spongiosa-fibrin-glue-plug

One 64-year-old male patient, with an 8-cm shaft defect of his tibia, required three spongiosa transplants before bridging of the defect was completed. The course of the post-operative state of infection, as documented by determination of ESR and WBC, is shown in Figs. 1 and 2. Compared with the values at the day of operation, both parameters had decreased significantly by the 2nd and 4th postoperative week respectively (P < 0.001).

Case Report

A 34-year-old diabetic and obese male patient showed signs of early infection following buttress plate (T-plate) osteosynthesis of his tibial head fracture. Intra-operatively, large parts of the bone underneath the plate were identified as necrotic. Removal of the plate and radical debridement left a large defect in the tibial head (Fig. 3) which was filled during a second operation with a spongiosa-fibrin-glue-plug. The fracture was temporarily stabilised by external fixation.

Scintigraphic examination 2 weeks following transplantation of spongiosa showed significant activity in the area of the transplant, as a sign of increased metabolism with hypervascularisation of the entire area. Four months later, the scintigraphic control showed only minor activity in the same area. Hence, the osteoclastic and osteoblastic processes, which had caused increased metabolism, may have been concluded approximately 4 months following the transplantation. The X-ray (Fig. 4) showed complete ossification of the former defect. This result is particularly noteworthy in the light of the patient's history of diabetes and his pronounced obesity of 120 kg bodyweight, both factors usually being associated with delayed wound healing.

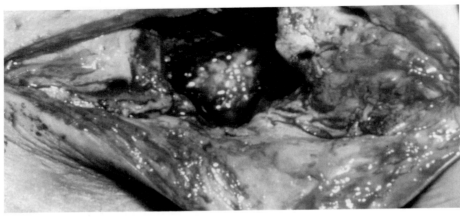

Fig. 3. Bone defect after radical debridement in a case of early infection of a tibial head osteosynthesis in a 34-year-old patient

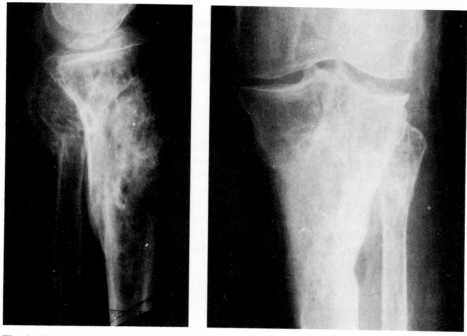

Fig. 4. The X-ray performed 4 months after spongiosa-fibrin-glue-plug shows complete ossification of the former defect

Discussion

The use of the spongiosa-fibrin-glue-plug for bridging and filling of bone shaft defects and cavities showed good results in our patients who suffered from post-traumatic or post-osteitic bone destruction. However, we do not believe that the addition of fibrin-glue to the spongiosa has a direct effect on its osteogenetic potency or promotes proliferation of blood vessels. The mechanism by which fibrin-glue may enhance early vascularisation may be seen in its ability to reduce micro-movements between the transplant and the surrounding tissue. A close contact between those two structures may be the basis for undisturbed proliferation of vessels into the transplant. Early vascularisation of the transplanted spongiosa is considered a prerequisite for the metabolic processes which lead to new bone formation.

In particular, septic cases in traumatology may be a domain for the use of fibrin-glue, since unfavourable wound conditions, insufficient blood supply, and a spongiosa-receiving bed of often dystrophic bone may impede primary healing of the implanted spongiosa. In these cases, the addition of fibrin-glue may improve the wound conditions. However, there is no doubt that adequate surgical debridement is imperative prior to the use of fibrin-glue as an adjuvant. Furthermore, the important role of the spongiosa itself should be emphasised. This is particularly important in view of the observation that the addition of too much fibrin-glue to the spongiosa may increase proliferation of fibroblasts to a point where in turn endothelial proliferation and callus formation may be impeded.

Hence, fibrin-glue may be a helpful adjuvant to enhance rebuilding of bone defects following trauma, and in particular, following septic complications, like osteitis.

Summary

The use of a spongiosa-fibrin-glue-plug for the bridging of post-traumatic bone defects in 102 patients is reported. The group consisted primarily of patients with large bone defects resulting from debridement in cases of post-traumatic osteitis. In 95% of the patients, only one operation was needed for sufficient reconstruction of the defect with the spongiosa-fibrin-glue-plug. Postoperative routine examinations showed that signs of infections as documented by ESR and WBC had subsided by the 2nd and 4th postoperative week, respectively. Therefore, we recommend the use of the spongiosa-fibrin-glue-plug for the treatment of large bone defects and for bridging of long shaft discontinuities.

References

1. Ascherl R, Geissdörfer K, Lechner F, Blümel G (1984) Fibrinklebung und kältekonservierte, homologe Spongiosa-Indikation, klinische Erfahrung und Ergebnisse beim Wiederholungseingriff in der Hüftgelenksendoprothedik. In: Fibrinklebung, J Scheele (Hrsg.), Springer Verlag Berlin Heidelberg New York, 214–220
2. Gerngross H, Claes L (1982) Der Einbau der autologen Fibrinkleberspongiosaplastik in das ersatzschwache und ersatzstarke Kortikalislager. In: Fibrinkleber in Orthopädie und Traumatologie, H. Cotta, A Braun (Hrsg.) G Thieme Verlag Stuttgart 75–78
3. Neugebauer R, Burri C, Ulrich Ch (1985) Funktionswiederherstellung durch simultane autologe Spongiosaplastik und Muskellappentransposition bei osteitischen Defekten an der unteren Extremität. In: Langenbeck Archiv Chirurgie 366:622
4. Rogge D, Kalbe P, Tizian C, Hock J (1985) Wiederherstellung großer Knochendefekte mit autogenen, allogenen und mikrovasculären gestielten Transplantagen. In: Langenbeck Archiv Chirurgie 366:662–663
5. Stübinger B, Fritsche H.-M, Erhardt W, Senekowitch R, Wuttke V, Blümel G (1982) Experimentelle Anwendung des Fibrinklebers zur Fixation cortico-spongiöser Fragmente und bei der autologen Spongiosaplastik. In: Fibrinkleber in Orthopädie und Traumatologie, H Cotta, A Braun (hrsg.) G Thieme Verlag Stuttgart 65–67
6. Wolf N, Scheele J, Link W, Beck H (1984) Die Spongiosaplastik beim Hüftgelenkersatz mittels zementfreier Judet-Prothesen. In: Fibrinklebung, J Scheele (hrsg.) Springer Verlag Berlin Heidelberg New York 211–213
7. Zilch H (1981) Der Einfluß des Fibrinklebers auf die Revaskularisierung des Knochentransplantates. In: Unfallheilkunde 84, 353–362

The Effect of Fibrin Sealant on Blood Flow and Bone Formation in Autologous Cancellous Bone Transplants: An Experimental Investigation in Dogs

U. Lucht, C. Bünger, J.T. Møller, F. Joyce, and H. Plenk Jr.

Key words: Autologous bone transplants, fibrin sealant, blood flow, bone formation, histomorphometry

Abstract

To study bone formation and regional blood flow after transplantation of autologous cancellous bone with and without the use of fibrin sealant (FS), iliac crest bone chips were filled into standardized tibial defects of 18 dogs, and only on one side the bone chips were mixed with FS while the other side served as control.

After 7, 14 and 21 days the regional blood flow was calculated from radiolabeled microsphere injections, and bone formation and remodeling were evaluated histomorphometrically.

In both sides, the highest blood flow rates were observed 14 days postoperatively. FS treatment did not significantly alter blood flow and new bone formation. In contrast, the fibrin clots at the surface of the graft inhibited the ongoing bone formation at 7 days post operation. Thus, FS treatment cannot be generally recommended for the transplantation of bone, but only as hemostatic agent and when transplants have to be kept in place, and then solely as a thin layer.

Introduction

The present study was carried out in order to contribute to the clarification of the role of fibrin sealant (FS) in bone transplantation. In an experimental model of autologous cancellous bone transplantation, the influence of FS was evaluated by regional blood flow measurements and estimation of new bone formation.

Material and Methods

Eighteen adult mongrel dogs (19-33 kg) were used. The FS was a two-component glue, (Immuno, Austria) for dogs. The anesthetized dogs were placed on their right or left side depending upon which hip was used as bone donor site and cancellous bone was taken from the iliac crest. The dogs were then placed in the supine position. A length-wise incision over the anterior tibia was made exposing the bone. An area of a length of 1.5 cm was marked on the middle of the tibia and a half cylinder of bone was removed (Fig.1). The bone marrow in the 1.5-cm-long area was removed and the central bone artery cauterized.

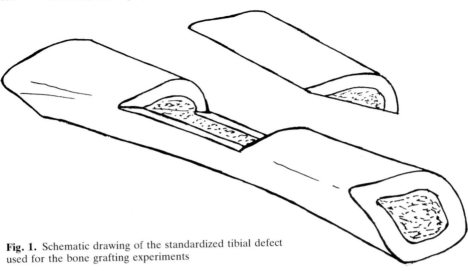

Fig. 1. Schematic drawing of the standardized tibial defect used for the bone grafting experiments

The cancellous bone from the iliac crest was kept in a dish at room temperature covered with isotonic saline-saturated gauze. Prior to use, the graft was divided into two parts and cut into chips. The two components of the FS (without aprotinin) were preheated to 37°C. Half of the chips were soaked with 1 ml of the mixed FS and after random allocation pressed into the tibial defect of the left or right side after which stability was ensured with an AO-plate.

The same procedure was performed on the contralateral leg, except that the cancellous bone was not treated with FS.

The dogs were divided into three groups and on the 7th, 14th and 21st postoperative day each of the three groups was analyzed by measurement of regional blood flow rates, histology and histomorphometry.

NEN-TRAC microspheres (New England Nuclear) with a diameter of 15 μm labeled with [113]Sn were used to measure the regional blood flow. The spheres were injected through a catheter in the left ventricle and reference blood sampling was taken from the abdominal aorta.

After flow measurements, the dogs were killed and the cancellous bone grafts were cut out and each divided into a superficial and a profound part of equal size. Then, the samples were placed in plastic vials with Schaffer's solution. Gamma radiation counting and calculation of regional blood flow rates were performed as described earlier (Bünger et al. 1983).

Undecalcified graft samples were embedded into methylmethacrylate; and tri-chrome-Goldner stain, toluidine blue, modified von Kossa stain and PAS-Alcian blue were applied. In addition, for the demonstration of fibrin, the phosphotungstic-acid-hematoxylin (PTAH) method was used. The trichrome-Goldner-stained sections were analyzed morphometrically and the following parameters were calculated: volume densities (%) of transplanted bone and newly formed mineralized bone and osteoid and surface densities (mm^2/mm^3) of newly formed bone and vessels in the marrow cavities. The surface densities of the new bone were divided into remodeling and resting bone.

Table 1. Blood flow rates in bone grafts (mm/min/100 g) (means ± SEMs)

		Day 7	Day 14	Day 21
Superficial	FS	17.92 ± 5.65	36.24 ± 9.81	12.05 ± 2.46
Bone graft	C	18.99 ± 7.55	33.61 ± 9.22	12.77 ± 1.31
Profound	FS	25.40 ± 7.61	32.99 ± 12.84	6.47 ± 0.66
Bone graft	C	22.28 ± 6.74	23.12 ± 7.23	9.74 ± 1.79
Total	FS	20.41 ± 7.03	34.80 ± 10.08	9.99 ± 1.72
Bone graft	C	20.37 ± 6.05	29.42 ± 8.35	11.22 ± 1.24

FS, side with fibrin adhesive system added to the graft; C, side of control

Mean values and standard error of the means (SEM) were calculated from the recorded parameters. Comparison of test and control values was performed by a paired t-test.

Results

Blood Flow Rates

Table 1 shows that the blood flow in the transplanted cancellous bone increased from the 7th to the 14th postoperative day, after which it decreased to reach the lowest level on the 21st day after operation. Comparison of the blood flow rates in the superficial bone grafts, the profound bone grafts as well as the total bone grafts showed no significant differences between FS-treated grafts and controls at any time.

Histology

Seven days after operation, new bone formation had started. However, in the superficial FS-treated grafts, many transplanted bone chips were still enveloped in fibrin clots (Fig. 2a) and showed no signs of cellular reaction or new bone formation. There was a clear borderline visible where cellular and vascular invasion had started into the fibrin clots, and below new bone formation was found (Fig. 2b). Small superficial fibrin clots were also observed in one of the controls but in this sample "normal" new bone formation was ongoing.

Fourteen days after operation, there was distinctly more newly formed bone and active remodeling in the superficial grafts of both groups (Fig. 2c). The grafted bone chips were always recognizable by their empty lacunae; and new bone formation, in some cases, filled the spaces between the chips. Bone formation started from either the surfaces of the bone chips or directly in the cell-rich, vascularized tissue in between. In some places, formations of hemopoietic cells could be seen around wide sinusoidal vessels. In the profound, FS-treated grafts, reactions seemed less pronounced than in the superficial, FS-treated grafts.

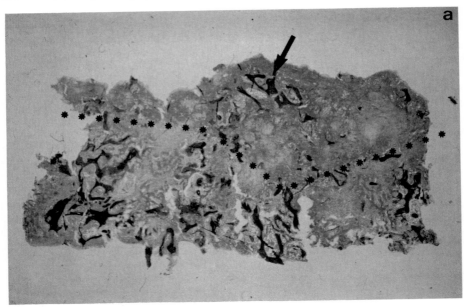

a

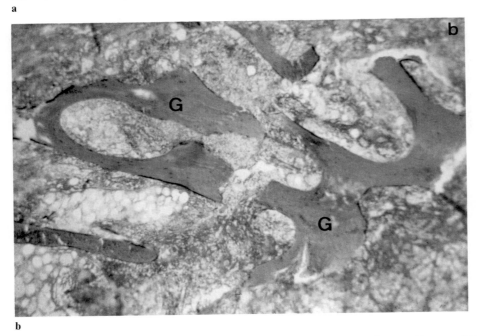

b

Fig. 2 a–c. Undecalcified microtome sections of the superficial portion of an FS-treated bone graft 7 days after operation. *a* Trichrome-Goldner stain, × 7; *b* PTAH-fibrin stain, × 110; *c* Trichrome-Goldner stain, × 110. *a* The outer area of the superficial graft (*above the asterisks*) is soaked with the fibrin sealant, and there *b* the grafted bone chips *(G)* show practically no reaction. *c* In the area below the asterisks, ongoing new bone formation (NB) can be seen around the vascularized granulation tissue and upon the surface of grafted bone chips *(GB)*

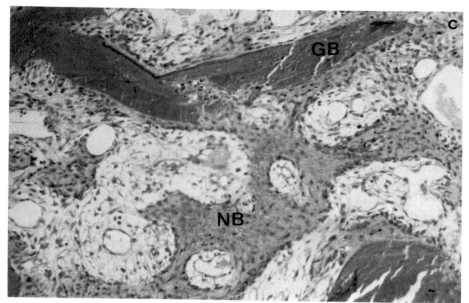

Fig. 2 c

Twenty-one days after operation, the bone samples from the superficial region seemed more dense, in some cases having a corticalis-like structure. The grafted bone chips were still recognizable but fully incorporated into new bone which showed mainly lamellar structure. A "tunneling resorption" of the grafted dead bone occurred in some places. In areas with less active remodeling, the marrow cavities were filled with hemopoietic marrow. There was no obvious difference between FS-treated and control grafts.

Histomorphometry

The volume density of grafted bone was very uniform in all the grafts examined. No significant difference between FS-treated grafts and controls was found.

Table 2. New bone volume density (%) (means ± SEMs)

		Day 7	Day 14	Day 21
Superficial	FS	6.72 ± 3.07	39.21 ± 7.28	28.18 ± 5.61
Bone graft	C	12.17 ± 4.22	30.54 ± 7.93	36.27 ± 2.23
Profound	FS	11.54 ± 3.99	14.05 ± 0.62	27.06 ± 3.49
Bone graft	C	11.43 ± 4.05	21.16 ± 7.63	27.07 ± 4.99
Total	FS	9.13 ± 2.50	26.63 ± 5.83	27.62 ± 1.65
Bone graft	C	11.80 ± 2.71	25.85 ± 5.39	31.67 ± 3.07

FS, side with fibrin adhesive system added to the bone graft; C, side of control

Table 3. New bone formation – surface density (mm^2/mm^3) (means ± SEMs)

		Day 7	Day 14	Day 21
Superficial	FS	1.61 ± 0.71	6.54 ± 0.53	4.56 ± 0.28
Bone graft	C	3.06 ± 1.09	5.40 ± 1.03	4.10 ± 0.51
Profound	FS	3.53 ± 1.14	2.69 ± 0.48	3.11 ± 0.80
Bone graft	C	3.59 ± 0.89	4.33 ± 1.67	3.28 ± 0.58
Total	FS	2.57 ± 0.72	4.57 ± 0.79	3.83 ± 0.48
Bone graft	C	3.32 ± 0.66	4.87 ± 0.93	3.69 ± 0.39

FS, side with fibrin adhesive system added to the bone graft; C, side of control

Seven days after the operation, there was a lower volume density (Table 2) and surface density (Table 3) of new bone formation in the superficial, FS-treated grafts compared with controls, but the differences were not significant. The same applied to the surface density of remodeling zones and vessels in the superficial graft. In the profound, FS-treated grafts and controls, the corresponding values were very uniform.

Fourteen days after operation, there was a trend toward diminished new bone formation, remodeling activity and surface density of vessels in the profound, FS-treated grafts compared with controls, but again the differences were not significant. In the superficial grafts, significant differences were not observed either.

Twenty-one days after operation, new bone formation, remodeling activity and surface density of vessels were equal in the FS-treated grafts and controls.

Discussion

In the present experimental model, the tibial blood supply was reduced by cauterization of the tibial artery in order to standardize the model but, simultaneously, to create suboptimal conditions as often seen in humans. The experimental model may, thus, be regarded as appropriate for the study of a possible favorable effect of FS.

The histological study showed that FS did not accelerate new bone formation. On the contrary, there was a tendency toward diminished bone formation in the FS-treated superficial bone grafts on the 7th day and the FS-treated profound grafts on the 14th day. On the 7th day, this may be explained by the observation that many of the transplanted bone chips were still surrounded by fibrin. The blood flow of the grafts was not affected by the FS-treatment but it should be emphasized that the increase of blood flow from the 7th to the 14th day coincided with increased bone formation in both FS and control groups.

These quantitative data are in contrast with previous reports of improved bone formation and accelerated vascularization as a result of FS-treatment (Arbes et al. 1981, Bösch 1981).

We have used the technique for bone grafting with FS as recommended by Bösch (1981). The chips with FS were pressed into the bone bed and excessive FS removed. Thus, the present model fulfills the demand for a thin layer of FS and there should be no impediment for the biological degradation of fibrin.

Conclusion

The present study, using a bone grafting technique similar to the technique used in humans, showed that FS had no favorable effect on bone vascularization and new bone formation in autologous cancellous bone grafts. Thus, there seems to be no indication for FS in ordinary transplantation of autologous cancellous bone. If used as a hemostatic agent, or as a glue in situations where it is difficult to keep the transplant in place, it should be applied in a thin layer.

References

1. Arbes H, Bösch P, Lintner F & Salzer M (1981). First clinical experience with heterologous cancellous bone grafting combined with the fibrin adhesive system. Arch Orthop Traumat Surg 98, 183-188
2. Bösch P (1981). Die Fibrinspongiosaplastik. Experimentelle Untersuchungen und klinische Erfahrung. Wr Klin Wschr 93, Suppl 124, 1-26
3. Bünger C, Hjermind J & Bülow J (1983). Hemodynamics of the juvenile knee in relation to increasing intra-articular pressure. Acta orthop scand 54, 80-87

Our Experience in Nerves, Tendon and Cartilage Sealing in more than 50 Cases

G. Krakovits and I. Tacsik

Key words: Fibrin sealing, reconstructive surgery, tendon, cartilage, nerves

Abstract

In the past 5 years we have performed over 50 fibrin sealings in cases of tendon, nerve and cartilage injury. Fibrin fixation of nerves and Achilles tendon gave an excellent result. Though all the cartilage fixations were effective, the healing process of the knee joint was less efficient.

Introduction

In Hungary fibrin sealant was first used by Vecsey (1980) in urological operative practice. We have used this method for 5 years in orthopaedic surgery, in the first 2 years very rarely, because of the fear of possible hepatitis virus infection and also because we were restricted by the relatively high cost of the material.

By courtesy of Immuno AG (Vienna) we were able to perform fibrin sealing in a total of 50 cases, which is a limited number compared with the 2500 operations a year in our department.

We very strictly followed all the instructions given by Spängler [5]. We performed all our operations when the wound was undoubtedly free from infection and always in closed, absolutely sterile air ventilation.

Methods and Results

We performed fibrin sealing in closed Achilles tendon rupture; in 6 cases within 24 h, in 5 cases within 48 h; two patients were operated on 10 and 20 days after the injury. The average age of the patients was 32 years.

We used three different types of operation; end-to-end anastomosis alone, anastomosis with the enforcement of the tendon plantaris, or anastomosis with plicating and bending down a 2×3-cm part of the proximal sheet of the triceps muscle. Rupp and Stemberger [3] published their experiences of tendon sealing with the aid of Z-suture, but we carried out all our tendon sealing – even when the tendon fibers were disarranged (Fig. 1a) – without suture (Fig. 1b). The average immobiliza-

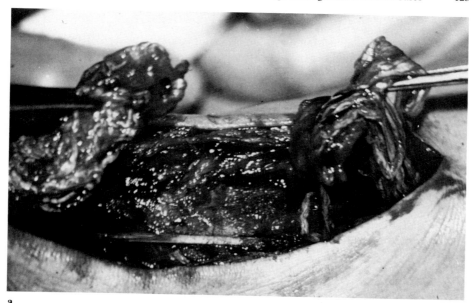

a

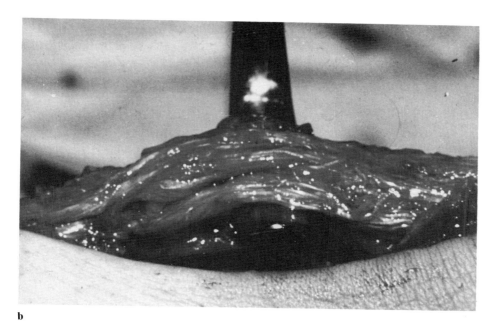

b

Fig. 1 a u. b. *a* Intraoperative picture of a ruptured Achilles tendon (46-year-old male) *b* After precise adaptation and fibrin sealant application, the tendon withstands strain

tion time in the walking cast was 5 weeks. The follow-up time in 6 cases was more than 3 years and more than 6 months in 7 cases.

There was no complication in wound healing during the follow-up time, no recurrent rupture, no limited movements and no complaints because pain occurred. Besides the regained range of normal motion there was no difference in the strength of plantar flexion between the operated and the normal side. All of them went back to work within 2 months.

The most favorable condition for healing of divided ligament is direct apposition of the surfaces. Such apposition minimizes scarring, accelerates repair, hastens collagenization and comes closer to restoring normal ligament tissue.

We attribute the excellent results which we present in Table 1, to the method by which such a close adaptation in such a large damaged area could be effected.

We used fibrin sealing for re- or transplantation of cartilage in five cases.

A 19-year-old boy suffered a direct trauma of the knee: a 2×2-cm piece was fractured off the condylar face of the patella (Fig.2a). The following day we replaced it with fibrin sealant (Fig. 2b). After 4 weeks in a walking cast and later on regular physiotherapy he was able to continue to play professional football.

In four cases (males) replantation was done on the condylar surface of the femur as Rupp and Stemberger [4] have described. In two cases we had to complete the replantation with a piece of cartilaginous bone gained from the neutral side of the femoral condyle. One patient was 50 years old, the other three less than 20. The follow-up time was more than 4 years (Table 2).

Table 1. Achilles tendon sealing

Operation Method	Number	Plaster cast	Function	Complication
Adaptation	8	5 weeks	Excellent	0
Adaptation + reinforcement with the plantaris tendon	3	5 weeks	Excellent	0
Adaptation + reinforcement with the musculus soleus flap	2	5 weeks	Good	0

Table 2. Replantation of cartilage-subchondral bone with fibrin sealant

	Number	Results		Complication
		Pain	Function	
Patella	1	0	Excellent	0
Femur condyle	4	1	Good	0

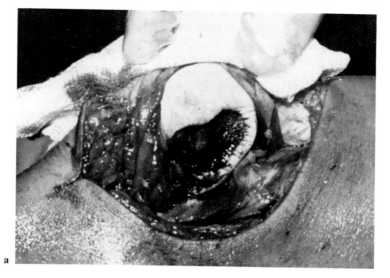

a

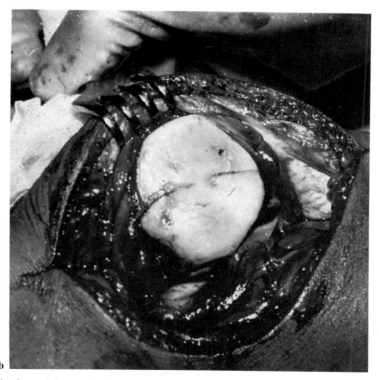

b

Fig. 2 a u. b. Condylar face of the patella shows the bed of the separated piece (23-year-old male) after a sports injury; *b* Replantation with fibrin sealant offers a very solid reinforcement

We estimated the result of transplantations on the loading areas as fairly good, compared with our experiences in the fracture clinic, e.g., removing only the fractured part or replacing it with pins or screws failed in all of our cases. The X-ray check up after 4 years showed no recurrent dislocation of the replantation though the clinical appearance was worse. All the four patients had complaints of swelling up of the joint and a certain pain during walking or standing. We do not want to discuss whether the cartilage replantation does promise success for the future but it was certain that the fibrin sealing served its original purpose: efficient fixation.

In two cases – outside our evaluation – we rubbed the femoral condyle of the damaged areas and mixed the cartilage mash with Tissucol and smeared it back, thus creating a film on the bone surface. After 2 months – 4 weeks unloaded walking in plaster cast-the two patients reported great improvement.

The elapsed time is too short to make a statement, and it would also require an arthroscopic examination.

In hand surgery we had excellent results with the volar nerve reconstructions. The operations were performed according to the method of Matras [1], 3 – 6 weeks after the first surgery.

On three occasions nerve sealing was done with adaptation of the nerves when the two injured ends could be approximated without any stretching. A plaster cast for 3 weeks was applied, the wrist in a bent position. The average age of the patients was 38 years. No complication in wound healing was seen.

We used fibrin sealant in 18 cases of nerve transplantation. The nervus suralis was excised and transplanted in the usual way. After sharp cutting the ends of the nerves at right angles – and precisely adapting them – we put the two adapted parts on an aluminum foil. After dropping fibrin sealant onto the anastomosis we rolled it over the nerve. Holding together the nerve fibers it prevents the sealant from getting between the ends and made a "cuff" around the anastomosis. This "cuff" keeps the ends so strong that we can lift them up with some force (Fig.3). After 3 weeks' immobilization of the arm in a cast, active exercises were started.

All the controls were done for more than 1 year; the cases were evaluated with respect to feelings of pain and heat, sweating [triketohydrindene (Ninhydrin) test] and sensibility according to Nicholson and Seddon [2]. The evaluations were in the range of 3-4 (Table 3).

Last but not least the method has an immense advantage by saving time for the surgeon: the operating time is decreased to half the usual time. The case number and control period of our study are not sufficient to give a definitive opinion but we are convinced that this method should not be absent from the arsenal of our medical weapons.

Table 3. Nerve sealing

Operation Method	Number	Plaster	Results			Complication
			Good	Fair	Poor	
Adaptation	3	3 weeks	2	1	0	0
Transplantation	18	3 weeks	10	5	3	0

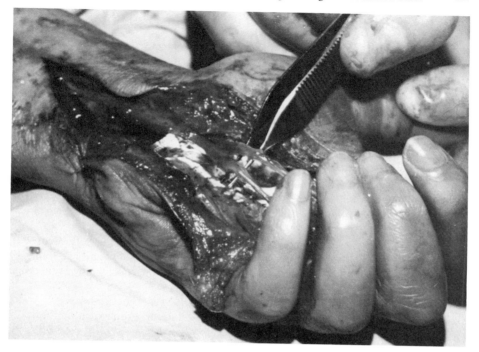

Fig. 3. After segment nerve transplantation the fibrin cuffs give strong resistance against mechanical stress

References

1. Matras H, Dinges H P, Mamoli B, Lassmann H (1973) Non-sutured nerve transplantation. J max-fac Surg 1: 37-40
2. Nicholson O R, Seddon H J (1957) Nerve repair in civil practice. Results of treatment of median and ulnar nerve lesions. Brit med J 2: 1065-1067
3. Rupp G, Stemberger A (1978) Versorgung frischer Achillesehnenrupturen mit resorbierbarem Nahtmaterial und Fibrinkleber. Med Welt 29: 796-798
4. Rupp G, Stemberger A (1978) Fibrinklebung in der Orthopaedie: Fixierung autologer Knorpel-Knochen-Wechsel-Plomben zur Wiederherstellung destruierter Kniegelenksknorpel. Med Welt 29: 766-767
5. Spängler H P (1976) Gewebeklebung und lokale Blutstillung mit Fibrinogen, Thrombin und Blutgerinnungsfaktor XIII. Wien Klin Wschr 88 Supp 49 1-18.
6. Vecsey D (1980) Tapasztalatok uj szövetragasztó anyag urológiai alkalmazásával. (Experiences with fibrin sealing in the urological practice). Orvosi Hetilap (Hungarian Medical Journal) 121: 1511-1515.

The Use of Fibrin Sealant (Tissucol/Tisseel) in Experimental and Clinical Traumatology

H. Kuś, H. Kędra, and J. Staniszewska-Kuś

Key words: bone implants, parenchymatous bleeding, peripheral nerves, tissue adhesives

Abstract

For 25 years we have tested almost all known tissue adhesives and have also used some of them in patients. We have found the fibrin adhesive Tissucol/Tisseel, (Immuno Austria) to be the best of all tissue adhesives in fulfilling biological and surgical requirements.

After some years of experimental and clinical trials we now use Tissucol with success and without complications in the following surgical indications: filling of large bone defects with bone grafts, skin transplants, and parenchymatous bleeding (liver, spleen).

The most controversial subject is the gluing of nerves. The authors give some examples of their own indications for such a procedure and their own methods.

Introduction

For 25 years we have been dealing in experimental, preclinical, and clinical studies on biomaterials. From the clinical point of view, biomaterials as implants may be divided into four groups:
1. Biostatic, biomechanical, and bioaesthetic implants and grafts
2. Materials for suture or tissue bonding (surgical sutures, tissue adhesives and bone cements)
3. Implants for direct contact with circulating blood
4. Artificial organs and their parts [5]

In the second group we have studied experimentally all known kinds of sutures and 15 types of tissue adhesive and analyzed their advantages and disadvantages. Sutures and ligatures have until now been the standard methods of surgical tissue repair. Highly developed suture materials have not always been sufficient to prevent complications. Granulomas and sutures cutting into parenchymatous organs or inflamed tissues are still phenomena of great practical importance. These factors as well as tissue ischemia and wound edge necrosis caused by sutures led to the development of various tissue sealants which originated from the basic desire for hemostasis of precapillary and capillary bleeding and at the same time atraumatic tissue repair.

Of many kinds of tissue adhesives, until 1980 we assigned only the butyl and isobutyl cyanoacrylates to limited clinical use [6]. In 1980 we began experimental and clinical studies using the fibrin sealant Human Immuno. This fibrin sealant

Fibrin Sealant in Operative Medicine
Traumatology and Orthopaedics – Vol. 7
Edited by G. Schlag, H. Redl
© Springer-Verlag Berlin Heidelberg 1986

proved to be the best from the biological point of view of all adhesives studied, as it caused the least tissue reaction, and the fibrinolysis could be controlled by proteinase inhibitors.

Although in our experimental studies a heterogenic material, defined as human fibrin adhesive, was used, it was possible to demonstrate many advantages of fibrin sealant, for instance in comparison with cyanoacrylates.

Methods and Results

In experimental studies first of all, we learned how to prepare and apply such adhesives and the limits of their clinical application. Experimental and pathomorphological studies were carried out on rats, rabbits, and piglets, to study the possibility of controlling bleeding from parenchymous organs (liver, spleen) and of tightening lung and tracheal tissue [10]. The absorption of fibrin sealant in soft and bone tissue during wound healing was also studied. Moreover, an experimental method for external sealing of preclotted vascular prostheses, implanted into the thoracic aorta in pigs, was worked out, utilizing a control device with disposable spray set for two-component fibrin sealant [2]. The experiments were carried out on over 300 animals (pigs, rabbits and rats).

The fibrin sealant Tissucol, after our experimental studies, was used clinically first for tightening pulmonary tissue and the sealing of suture lines on the tracheal and bronchial stumps after pneumonectomy and lobectomy, with good clinical results [10].

Another very important indication is the use of fibrin sealant for fixation of bone implants, mainly in filling large bone defects. It provides not only fixation of the bone graft, but also may stimulate the process of osteogenesis [1]. We have never encountered any adverse results of such a procedure: on the other hand, we often regretted its nonapplication.

There are also clinical indications, in traumatology, for the use of fibrin sealant in cartilage and skin graft fixation; however, our clinical experience in such cases is small to date.

We have also studied the use of fibrin sealant in surgical reconstruction and gluing of peripheral nerves [3-9]. This is the most controversial subject.

After several years of our own experimental and clinical studies, we think that fibrin sealant may be successfully used in the following clinical indications:
1. For complementary direct union of nerve fascicles, after our own method [3-4] (Fig. 1).
2. In cases of numerous nerve grafts, a single surgical suture, combined with fibrin sealant may extensively shorten the length of the operation and give similar results to those obtained after two to three, microsurgical adapting sutures [7] (Fig. 2).
3. Partial lesions of peripheral nerves [4] (Fig. 3).
4. In reconstruction of monofascicular nerve defects the use of one-bundle nerve grafts may be indicated, bonded at the ends by fibrin sealant only, and then sutured with the nerve stumps. In this way, we have achieved good clinical results (Fig. 4).

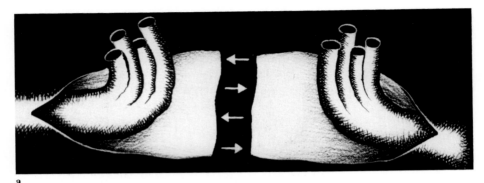

a

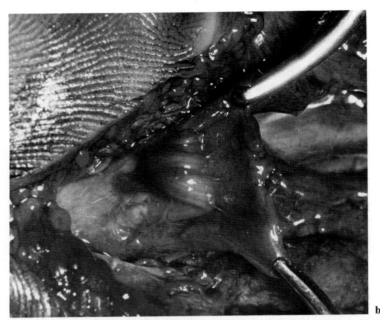

b

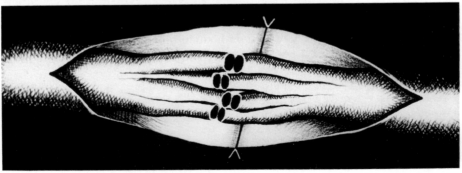

c

Fig. 1 a–c. Own method of direct nerve suture. *a* Schema of the method. *b* The epineurium prepared for the relaxation suture. *c* Nerve fascicles or their groups to be connected by sutures or fibrin adhesives

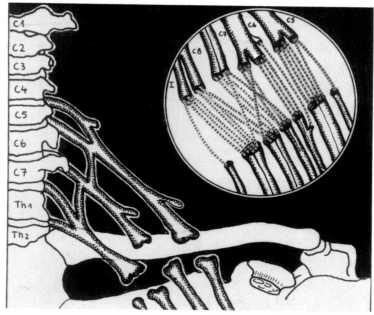

Fig. 2. Difficult and long-lasting reconstruction of nerves. *Example:* A total disruption of the brachial plexus. 24 sural nerve grafts were used and united to the plexus under the microscope. We used 48 single 10/0 sutures and additionally Tissucol, which facilitated the proper reconstruction of the brachial plexus. After 2 years a good clinical result was obtained

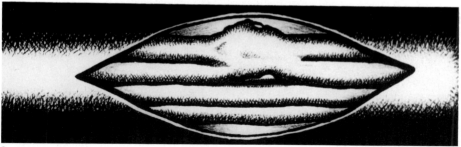

a

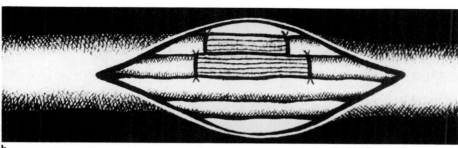

b

Fig. 3a u. b. Partial lesions of peripheral nerves may also be an indication for the use of fibrin sealant. *a* Neuroma of two fascicle groups after a direct lesion. *b* Reconstruction with nerve grafts may be done using fine sutures or simple fibrin adhesives

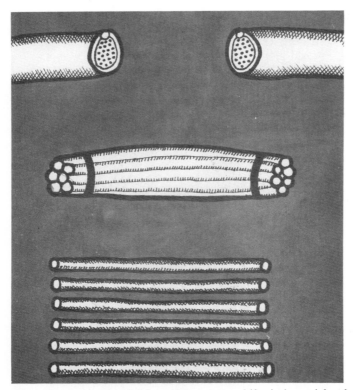

Fig. 4. Reconstruction of defects of mono- or multifascicular peripheral nerves may be done using the following procedure: five to eight sural nerve grafts are bonded at the ends by fibrin sealant and then sutured to refreshed nerve stumps

In the above-described trials we used very small amounts of fibrin sealant, which is put on nerve tissue with fine needles. For economy, reconstruction of peripheral nerves is performed simultaneously on two to four patients during the same day.

References

1. Orthopädie und Traumatologie (1982) 4. Heidelberger Orthopädie-Symposium, G Thieme Verlag, Stuttgart-New York
2. Kędra H, Rutowski R, Smetanski K, Solski L (1985) Zastosowanie kleju fibrynowego do uszczelniania protez naczyniowych. Wstępne badania doświadczalne. (The use of fibrin adhesive for sealing vascular prostheses. Preliminary experimental studies.) VII Konferencja-Biocybernetyka i Inżynieria Biomedyczna, Gdańsk 359-362
3. Kuś H (1983) Mikrochirurgische faszikuläre Nervennaht. Eigene Methode. Handchirurgie, Mikrochirurgie, Plastische Chirurgie 15:235
4. Kuś H (1984) Microsurgical reconstruction of peripheral nerves. Own experience. In Handbook of Microsurgery, CRC Press, Boca Raton, Florida

5. Kuś H (1985) Przeszczepianie tkanek i stosowanie elementów aloplastycznych. (Tissue transplants and alloplasty.) In: Traumatologia narządu ruchu, T.I. (Traumatology of the kinetic organs, vol I). PZWL Warszawa, 479-497
6. Kuś H, Kędra H: , Nervenanastomosen mit Fibrinklebung. Bericht über eigene Methode. Tagung "Die Anwendung von Klebern in der Medizin", Leipzig, (5-6 November 1982)
7. Kuś H, Rutowski R, Zarzycki A (1983) Badania nad doskonaleniem metod rekonstrukcji nerwów obwodowych. (Investigations on the improvement of methods of peripheral nerve reconstruction.) Polish Hand Surgery, 19, 1, 35
8. Kuś H, Araszkiewicz H (1984) Rekonstruktive Eingriffe am Plexus brachialis. Plastische und wiederherstellende Massnahmen bei Unfallverletzungen. Springer-Verlag, Berlin-Heidelberg
9. Kuś H, Kędra H 1984, Kliniczne zastosowanie kleju fibrynowego w mikrochirurgicznej rekonstrukcji nerwów obwodowych. (Clinical application of fibrin adhesive in microsurgical reconstruction of peripheral nerves.) Prace Naukowe Akademii Medycznej we Wrocławiu XVII, 2, 161-175, PWN, Warszawa-Wrocław
10. Rogalski E, Kędra H, Kuś H, Rogalski P (1985) Kleje fibrynowe. Wstępne badania doświadczalne i kliniczne (50 Jubilec Congress of Polish Surgeons, Kraków 1980). Polski Przeg Chir 1985. (Fibrin adhesives. First experimental and clinical studies.) Pol Przeg Chir I.57, nr1, 62-64

The Use of Fibrin Sealant in the Closure of Skin and Bone Defects in the Tibial Area After Third-Degree Open Fracture with Delayed Healing

K. Sandner and H. Arzinger-Jonasch

Key words: Skin and bone defects in the frontal tibial area, third-degree open lower leg fractures, delayed healing, closure of defects with fibrin sealant and epidermis patches, fibrinoblast-stimulating effect, factor XIII

Abstract

In third-degree open lower leg fractures with delayed healing, the closure of skin and bone defects in the frontal tibial area often causes considerable problems. A valuable and complementary contribution is made in the sealing of these defects by a mixture of fibrin sealant and epidermis patches, using the hemostatic, adhesive and wound-healing enhancing effect of fibrin sealant.

Introduction

The traumatologist is often faced with serious problems because of the considerable traumatization of the soft part structures and the bone in third-degree open lower leg fractures. The thin soft part coating in the area of the frontal tibial part, the difficult circulatory conditions and the often complicated fracture types demand a clear therapeutic concept and a professional wound toilet and first dressing. In spite of careful wound toilet, correctly performed debridement and early stable osteosynthesis, complications such as delayed wound healing or infections cannot always be prevented.

The international literature indicates an infection rate of up to 38% in third-degree open lower leg fractures; in our own patients we had an infection rate of 4.5% in all lower leg fractures. The secondary closure of skin and bone defects in the frontal tibial area is extremely difficult in the case of vascular and circulatory defects, or if the osteosynthesis material is partially open in the case of delayed wound healing. Numerous surgical methods are at our disposal for the closure of skin and bone defects in the lower leg area (see Table 1): Autologous split-thickness skin grafts (mesh-graft 1:1.5 or 1:3) are only successful if applied on suitable (fresh, clean granulation) and not infected wound bed. Shift grafts and rotatory grafts are of only limited use as contact grafts in the lower leg area. Muscle and myocutaneous grafts are simple and safe methods; however, they cannot be applied in the distal lower leg area. Cross-leg plasty is a good method to close larger defects with skin and subcutis by a distant flap; it necessitates, however, the fixation of the legs in an uncomfortable position for at least 3 weeks. Cross-leg plasty does not improve the vascularization of the graft bed, as the graft is supplied by vessels in the

Table 1. Surgical measures to close skin and bone defects in the lower leg area

1. Split-thickness skin graft
2. Contact grafts
   a) Shift grafts and rotatory grafts
   b) Muscle and myocutaneous flaps
3. Distant flaps
   a) Cross-leg plasty
   b) So-called wide flap
4. Microvascular tissue transfer

wound bed. The so-called "wide flap" requires immobilization of the limbs by external fixation for 3–4 weeks as well. In microvascular tissue transfer the musculus latissimus dorsi flap plays the most important role. Prerequisites for successful tissue transfer are the preoperative description of the vessels by angiography and a team of surgeons with experience in microsurgery and adequate equipment.

At the symposium on fibrin sealant held in 1982 at the Karl Marx University in Leipzig, Rupp reported on the successful application of fibrin sealant in wound healing. Rupp managed to close ulcera cruris, delayed healing wounds and skin defects at least temporarily with a mash of fibrin sealant and epithelium scratched from healthy skin parts. This biological wound dressing protected the bone and tendinous tissue underneath from dehydration. In ulcera cruris and badly healing wounds Rupp injected the components of the fibrin sealant into the wound edges. Hauser [3] confirmed the excellent results achieved by Rupp with fibrin sealant in the treatment of chronic wounds with poor healing prospects.

Material and Method

Encouraged by the promising application of fibrin sealant in wound healing in 1982 we started to seal skin and bone defects in the frontal tibial area after third-degree open lower leg fractures with delayed wound healing with a mixture of fibrin sealant (Tissucol) and epidermis patches taken from healthy skin parts. The epidermis patches are obtained from a very thin autologous split-thickness skin graft removed with an electrodermatome according to Mollowitz by mechanical cutting. They trigger the so-called "Reverdin effect". The interpretation of the mechanism of action is based on in vitro scientific experiments with fibroblasts by Bruhn et al. [1] and Turowski et al. [5]. They proved that fibrin sealant contains the substances thrombin, fibronectin, factor XIII and fibrin with a stimulating effect on fibroblasts. Factor XIII also accelerates the growth of granulation tissue and thus induces the reparative stage of wound healing.

The artificially produced wound crust represents a biological bandage that protects the tissue underneath from dehydration and mechanical influences. So far we have treated 12 patients with this method. We chose four patients to demonstrate our procedure.

Case 1 (B. D.)

This 30-year-old patient suffered a third-degree open lower leg fracture in a traffic accident, with a skin defect as large as a palm and considerable muscle crushing. In spite of immediate and exact wound debridement and stabilization of the fracture by an eight hole DC plate (dynamic compression plate), new muscle necroses appeared because of secondary vascular thromboses that had to be removed in a re-operation. The skin defect was closed with an autologous split-thickness mesh graft.

We were not able to prevent local soft tissue infection with formation of circumscribed osteitis. In spite of the skin defect and the infection osseous consolidation of the fracture took place. In 1983 the osteosynthesis material was removed and the infected skin and bone defect of 3×5 cm in the frontal tibial area were closed with a mash of fibrin sealant and epidermis patches. There were no complications in the further course of the disease; the local and functional results were excellent.

Case 2 (D. D.)

This 20-year-old patient suffered a multitrauma in a traffic accident with a motorcycle. The third-degree open lower leg fracture with a skin defect of 5×5 cm in the frontal tibial area was primarily stabilized by a seven-hole DC plate. Wound healing was delayed with formation of chronic osteitis because of a craniocerebral trauma that caused strong motoric agitation of the patient for a few days. Chronic osteitis required radical debridement; instability required a change in the osteosynthesis procedure. The fracture was immobilized by external fixation, the osteitis cavity filled with a gentamycin-PMMA chain (polymethylmethacrylate). After the infection was stopped the closure of the large skin and bone defect in the frontal tibial area was extremely difficult. The bone defect was closed with autologous spongiosa from the iliac crest in addition to fibrin sealant and gentamycin (fibrin-antibiotics combination) and an autologous split-thickness mesh skin graft. There were no further complications. Osseous consolidation of the fracture took place with maximum load capacity of the leg.

Case 3 (M. I.)

In a car accident this 59-year-old patient suffered a third-degree open proximal lower leg fracture at the left extremity (multiple fragment fracture with numerous small fragments) with extensive soft tissue contusion and a second-degree open supra- and intercondylar fracture of the femur. The fracture of the femur was stabilized by a 12-hole-condyle-support plate (Burri plate); the lower leg fracture was stabilized with an eight-hole T-plate and Kirschner's wire. For osteosynthesis only stabilization of the positioning was achieved because of the fracture and osteoporosis. Extensive soft tissue necroses appeared secondarily in the lower leg area with formation of chronic osteitis and sequestration. After radical debridement and sequestrotomy the remaining defect was filled with autologous spongiosa from the iliac crest. In spite of the partially open osteosynthesis plate osseous healing of the fracture took place. The remaining skin defect of 4.5 × 5.5 cm after the removal of material immediately beneath the tuberositas tibiae was closed with a mash of fibrin sealant and epidermis patches. After healing without complications the cosmetic and functional result was good.

Case 4 (R. A.)

In a typical rear end collision (bumper injury) with a motorcycle this 18-year-old patient suffered a third-degree open lower leg fracture with a large defect of substance of the fibula. The injured leg suffered a simultaneous arterial circulation disorder. The bone fracture was primarily stabilized by a nine-hole DC plate and a traction screw. The wound in the tibial area remained open and was covered with SYSpur-derm (temporary synthetic skin replacement made of polyesterpolyol and toluylendiisocyanat; product of the GDR), which guaranteed tension-free wound closure in the tibial area. Contusion marks caused by the accident in the frontal tibial area indicated the impending disaster a few days later. The contusion area became necrotic and had to be removed by surgery. After necrectomy a large part of the tibia was open. Dehydration of the uncovered bone could not be prevented even by covering the area with moistened SYSpur-derm several times a day. So we soon decided to close the existing skin defect with a mash of fibrin sealant and epidermis patches in the bone part and with split-thickness mesh grafts in the soft tissue part (Fig. 1). This measure prevented secondary bone necrosis. We were forced to remove the material and change the osteosynthesis procedure later because of chronic osteitis with instability (Fig. 2). With stabilization of the fracture by external fixation (three-dimensional) and autologous spongiosa transplantation osseous healing of the fracture took place. The leg has a maximum load capacity and is easily movable (Fig. 3).

Discussion

We can confirm the good results of fibrin sealant in wound treatment achieved by Rupp and Hauser. Compared with the methods for closing skin and bone defects in the lower leg area that are summarized in Table 1, fibrin sealing has the following advantages:
1. Easy to handle
2. May be applied at any time without technical expenditure
3. May be repeated several times
4. Guarantees at least temporary complete wound sealing
5. Protects bones and tendinous tissue from dehydration
6. Maintains the wound area almost aseptic for eventual plastic surgery

This method is a valuable and complementary contribution to the closure of skin and bone defects in the frontal tibial area after third-degree open lower leg fractures with delayed healing.

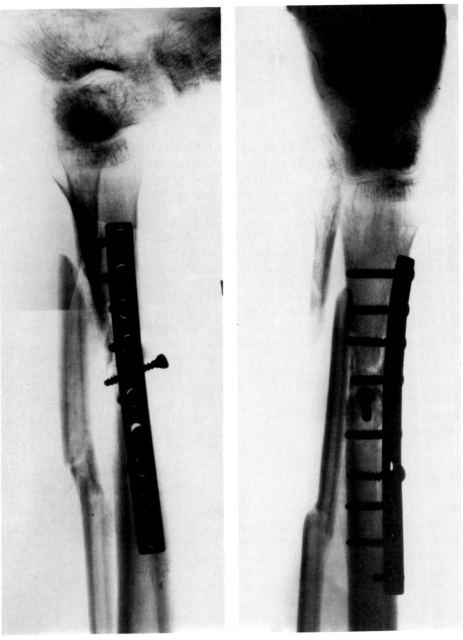

a   b

Fig. 1 a, b. Condition after third-degree open lower leg fracture, primarily managed by a nine-hole DC plate (dynamic compression plate) and surgical application of a traction screw. *c* Necrosis of a contusion area in the frontal tibial area. After necrectomy the tibia bone is partially uncovered. *d* Wound closure by a mash of fibrin sealant (Tissucol) and epidermis patches with additional autologous split-thickness mesh graft. *e* Secondary bone necrosis was prevented by wound sealing with fibrin sealant and epidermis patches

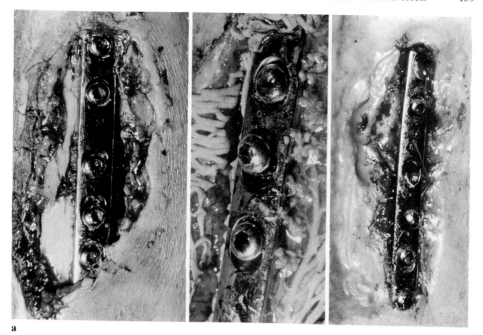

a

b

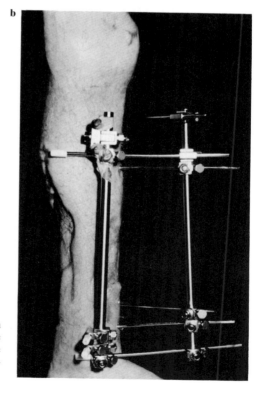

Fig. 2 a–c. Chronic osteitis with instability in the fractured area forced us to change the osteosynthesis procedure. Stabilization of the fracture by external fixation (three-dimensional).

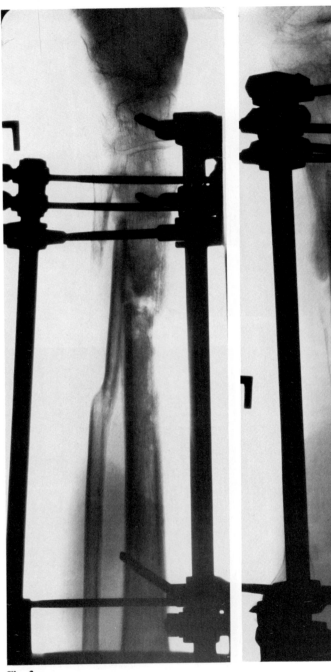
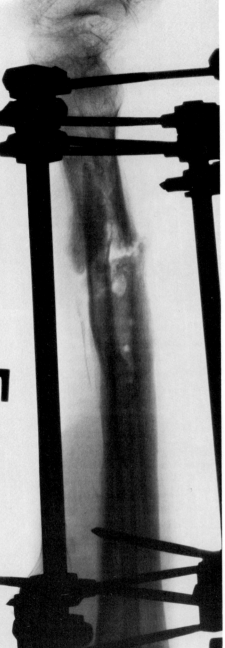

Fig. 2 c

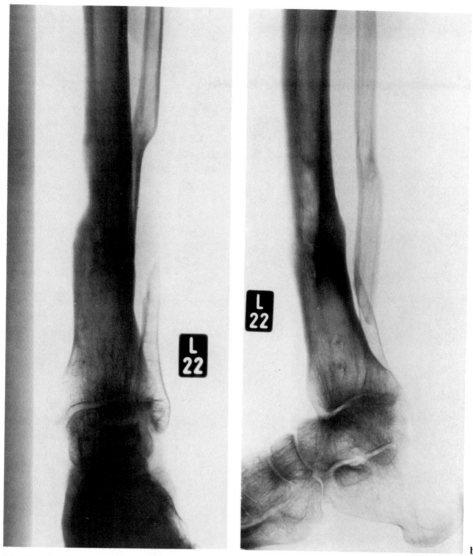

a
b

Fig. 3a u. b. Osseous consolidation of the fracture by means of external fixation and autologous spongiosa grafting after 9 months. *c, d* Maximum load capacity and good functioning of the leg

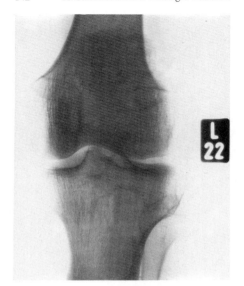
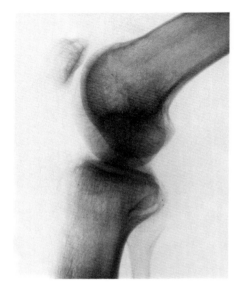
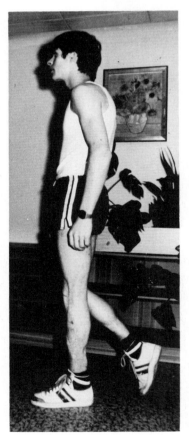
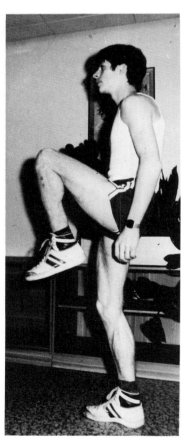

References

1. Bruhn HD, Christophers E, Pohl J, Scholl G (1980) Regulation der Fibroblastenproliferation durch Fibrinogen, Fibrin, Fibronektin und Faktor XIII, In: Schimpf K: Fibrinogen, Fibrin und Fibrinkleber Schattauer, 217–226
2. Egkher E, Spängler H (1983) Fibrinklebung in der operativen Medizin. 3.4. Traumatologie, edition medizin, Weinheim Deerfield Beach, Florida, Basel 71–85
3. Hauser J (1983) Der Fibrinkleber Tissucol® in der allgemeinen Chirurgie und Traumatologie, Symposium Sion, 18–39
4. Rupp G (1981) Traumatologie, Fixierung von Knorpel. Scient. Workshop Graz, 57–59
5. Turowski G, Schaadt M, Barthels M, Diehl V, Poliwoda H (1980) Unterschiedlicher Einfluß von Fibrinogen und Faktor XIII auf das Wachstum von Primär- und Kulturfibroblasten. In: Schimpf K: Fibrinogen, Fibrin und Fibrinkleber Schattauer, 227–237

Indications and Limits of Fibrin Adhesive Applied to Traumatological Patients

E. Egkher, H. Spängler, and H. P. Spängler

Key words: Fibrin adhesive, osteosynthesis, cartilage injury, parenchyma injury, skin transplantation, adhesive strength

Abstract

Optimal treatment of severe injuries of the bones consisting of very small fragments is frequently impossible with the usual means of osteosynthesis. If there is, additionally, damage of the joint including injuries of the cartilage and loss of the subchondral bony tissue the healing of this injury – healing which must be congruent with the joint – will be extremely successful with the help of fibrin adhesive. Very small fragments are put together by means of the adhesive and are inserted afterwards into the damaged part, in some cases even without using osteosynthesis.

We also regularly use this fibrin adhesive in the case of injuries of the tendon especially in the case of a rupture of the Achilles tendon. In contrast to different authors, we insert a sunk suture to repair and maintain the exact length of the tendon. Having exactly repaired the length the single bundles of fasciculi are glued to each other successively. Surplus tendon tissues are excised to give an optimal function of the tendon. In these cases not the maximum tensile stress to which the adhesive is subjected is decisive but the effect of the fibrin on the tissue in the bradytrophic tissue.

One area of application of the adhesive is its blood-staunching effect in the field of accident surgery. Severe contusions and ruptures of parenchymatous organs usually occur together with an enormous loss of blood and the destruction of the organ. Extensive foci of contusion in the brain can be sealed with the adhesive without further destruction of the organ. Large-scale injuries of the liver are closed by applying the adhesive. Prompt interruption of the areal bleeding is the consequence. Even the preservation of organs in the case of a rupture of the spleen is successful with this method.

Finally the covering of skin lesions should be mentioned. Deep recesses and wrinkles on the skin can be successfully treated by transplantation of skin only since the introduction of this adhesive.

Introduction

The high demands made on a biological adhesive in surgery cannot be satisfactorily met by the fibrin adhesive in all cases of traumatology. The extraordinary biological compatibility, a rapid haemostatic effect, also when extensive injuries of the tissue are involved, lack of toxicity, induction of the repair of the tissue and good elasticity enable the adhesive to maintain and seal defects; its stability as an adhesive, however, should not be overestimated especially with regard to the reabsorption, which frequently takes place too quickly. If we can assume that the injury will soon be properly supported with vessels, the exclusive application of the adhesive is mostly sufficient, unless the site of sealing is subject to excessive tensile stress. If bradytrophic tissue is involved and great permanent stress must be expected, further precautions for fixing and stabilizing must be taken [2, 3, 4, 5]. Disappointments occurring in traumatology when using our adhesive must frequently be traced back to the non-observance of these experiences. These disappointments might unjustly discredit the adhesive.

We would like to demonstrate in detail the indications and limitations of fibrin adhesive based on our experience in the treatment of traumatized patients.

As the technique of successful treatment, the results and problems of fibrin adhesion are different with regard to injuries of various organs and tissues, the results will be discussed in the corresponding sections immediately after the case description.

Parenchymatous Organs

In 1973 we used the adhesive for the first time in an emergency who had sustained an intensively bleeding, multiple rupture of the liver. After transfusion the severely injured patient suffered from a coagulation disorder so the bleeding from the large-scale injuries of the liver could not be stopped by sutures alone. Past experience has shown that the treatment of injured parenchymatous organs is one of the most important areas of application for fibrin adhesive in traumatology. In spite of the excessive proteolytic activity of these tissues, safe healing can be expected, due to the quick proliferation of tissue and vessels. Our experiments with pigs have definitely demonstrated that standardized inflicted injuries of the liver, spleen and pancreas heal quickly and without complications, leaving small scars (Fig. 1a–f). These experiments were carried out without additional supporting sutures. As in the case of a rupture of human organs large zones are usually heavily destroyed, the stability of the adhesive is consequently insufficient; central sutures are indispensable [4].

In addition to the heavy bleeding of ruptures of the liver the complications of abscess formation, biliaemia, and haemobilia should be pointed out. As it is possible to close large injuries of the liver especially when using a spray, even the smallest bile ducts can be closed, too. In this way, the possibility of an entry of bile into the abdomen and the bloodstream is avoided.

Results in recent scientific research [6] have shown that an organ-saving surgical intervention should be aimed at by all means in the case of injuries of the spleen, above all if children are involved. It has been pointed out several times that the fibrin adhesive in this case, too, is a useful method of successfully preserving this plethoric organ. We insist on intensive postoperative control and supervision if necessary by angiography and ultrasonography to discover postoperative haemorrhage in time.

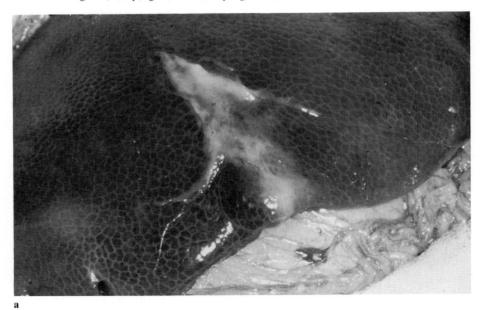

a

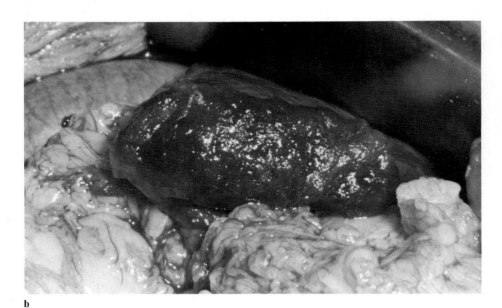

b

Fig. 1 a–f. The method of fibrin adhesive in the liver, the spleen and the pancreas of a pig *a–f*
Histology of scars

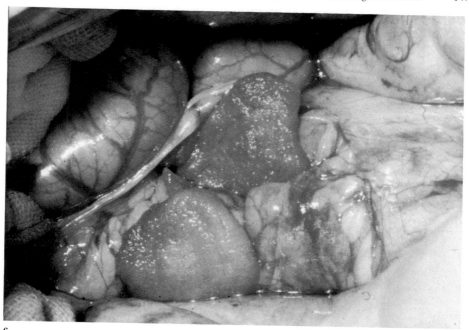

c

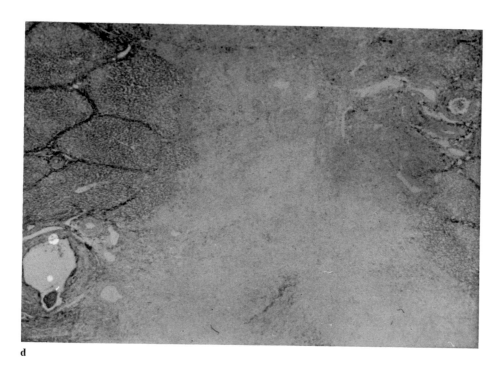

d

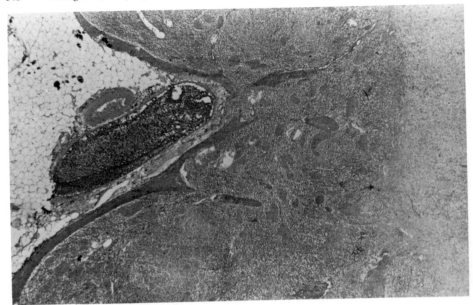

Fig. 1 e

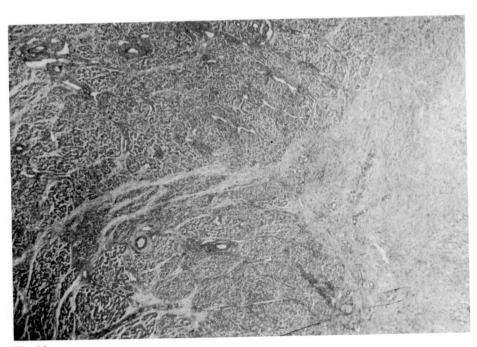

Fig. 1 f

As the solidity of the fibrin adhesive is insufficient to stabilize bone fragments a complete immobilisation (plaster cast, fixateur externe) is necessary. Only in exceptional cases involving small joints can this immobilisation be dispensed with.

As experiments have shown, even rare injury of the pancreas can be treated directly with the help of the adhesive. It will hardly be necessary to emphasize that drainage to avoid tryptic damage of the tissue. In the case of a severe renal injury, too, the organ may be saved with the help of the adhesive; an exact function test of the contralateral kidney is not always possible in a badly injured patient [7].

When injuries of the thorax make surgical intervention necessary, the adhesive, on account of its elasticity is compliant with the breathing excursion of the lungs. Nevertheless, we advise to treat deep injuries including ruptures of the bronchial tubes and vessels at first, and to apply the sealant when the lungs are inflated.

Skin

The fibrin adhesive can unreservedly be seen as the optimum method for skin transplantation. The skin transplant can be adapted extremely well to the surface without additional means only with the help of the fibrin adhesive even when large-scale furrows and recesses occur. Furthermore, a considerably quicker revascularization can be expected. These transplantations are well supplied with blood already after 3 days.

Bones

With regard to the formation of pseudarthrosis the healing of spongiosa transplants depends primarily on the intensity of blood supply in the transplant, on the amount and quality of the osteogenetic substance, and on the contact of the spongiosa with an area which is rich in vessels. If the spongiosa can only be implanted in an area of deficient blood supply, union with the vascular system which is of vital importance for graft take, is promoted by the sealant. The rate of integration can be considerably improved even in case of a heterological transplantation[1]. Multiple bone injuries in the region of the joint, consisting of small fragments, cannot be treated successfully with the common methods of osteosynthesis as this might cause additional damage. In this case we apply the following method: first of all, we stick together the smallest parts with the adhesive to rebuild the congruence of the joint. Then these larger fragments are stabilized together with the other parts as normal (Fig. 4).

This paper illustrates our experience with fibrin adhesive, which has proved quite satisfactory in our clinic for more than 12 years; on the other hand it has shown that this method can become discredited in the case of wrong indication, improper application, and overestimation of its adhesive power.

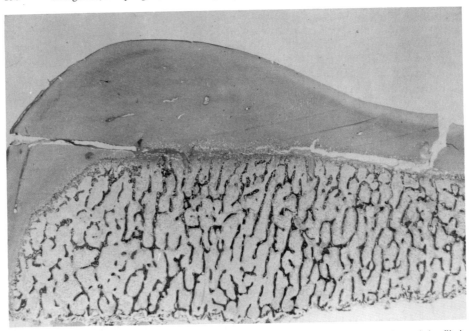

Fig. 2. Histology of a pure cartilage transplantation 10 days after operation. Vestiges of the fibrin adhesive can be seen only in the centre; it has been dissolved on the edges. Histology Plenk

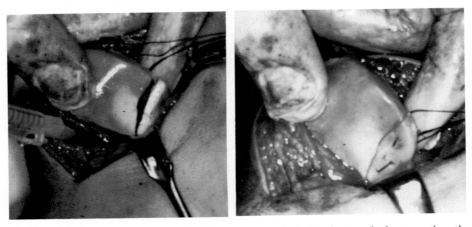

Fig. 3 a, b. Method of the replantation (suture and sealing) of a large-scale fracture when the cartilage of the knee joint is damaged. The replanted cartilage of this 12-year-old boy is without abnormal findings 2 years after the operation

Cartilage and Tendons

A quick process of reparation cannot be expected in the tissue of cartilages and tendons. Furthermore, tensile stress is usually great. Especially when cartilages are glued the fibrin adhesive cannot regenerate the tissue as quickly as fibrinolysis breaks it down. This fact is impressively demonstrated by our experimental studies in calves (Fig. 2). If the tensile stress acting on the cartillage cannot be avoided, for instance due to an unfavourable location, additional fixation is necessary (Fig. 3 a, b). Consequently, in addition to our adhesive we use a central supporting suture when repairing rupture of an Achilles tendon. Basically, a complete rehabilitation of this large tendon can only be obtained by an exact restoration of the tendon's length in order to reach the original strength for stretching.

We have found that this can be done with the above-mentioned technique. Sixteen ruptures of the Achilles tendon, treated recently with this combined method, led neither to healing complications nor to damage of various functions.

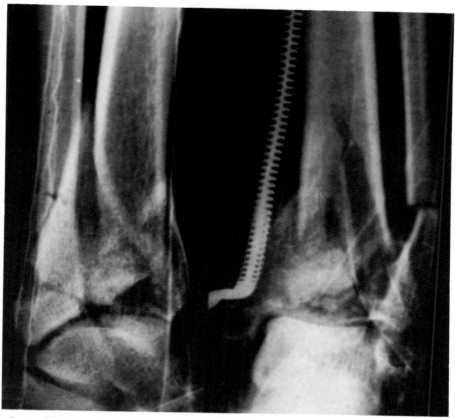

Fig. 4 a–c. *a* Heavily comminuted fracture with fragments of the distal tibia *b* treated with the fibrin adhesive and screws *c* and healing after the removal of the osteosynthesis material

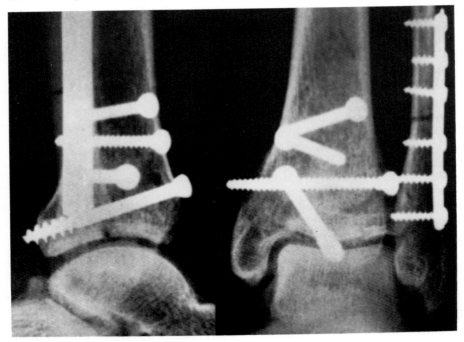

Fig. 4 b

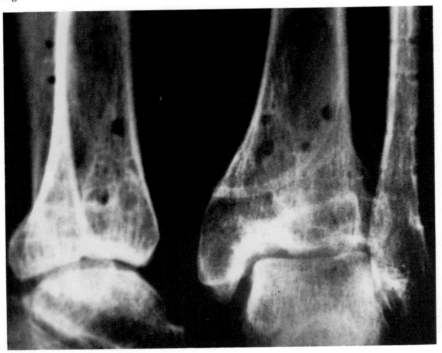

Fig. 4 c

References

1. Bösch P, Lintner F, Arbes H, Brand G (1980) Experimental investigations of the effect of the fibrin adhesive on the Kiel heterologous bone graft. Arch Orthop Traum Surg 96: 177
2. Claes L, Burri C, Helbing G, Lehner E (1982) Die Festigkeit von Knorpelklebungen in vitro. Fibrinkleber in Orthopädie und Traumatologie, Georg Thieme Verlag Stuttgart – New York 106
3. Edinger D, Mühling J, Schröder F, Will Ch, Heine WD (1983) Experimentelle Klebung von Vollhauttransplantaten. Fibrinkleber in Orthopädie und Traumatologie, Georg Thieme Verlag Stuttgart – New York 210
4. Egkher E, Spängler H (1983) Die Fibrinklebung in der operativen Medizin, Weinheim, Basel 71
5. Haas S, Stemberger A, Duspiva W, Ippisch A, Weidringer JW, Blümel G (1982) Zur Frage des Inhibitorzusatzes bei der Fibrinklebung, Fibrinkleber in Orthopädie und Traumatologie, Georg Thieme Verlag Stuttgart – New York 22
6. Passl R, Eibl M, Egkher E (1978) Immunologische Untersuchungen nach Splenektomie im Kindesalter aus traumatischer Ursache, Zbl Chirurgie 103, 560
7. Urlesberger H, Rauchenwald K, Henning K (1979) Fibrin adhesives in surgery of the renal parenchyma, Eur Urol 5, 260

Fibrin Sealant (Tissucol/Tisseel) in Emergency Surgery

U. Mercati, G. Antonini, and G. Castagnoli

Key words: Seals in emergency surgery, Tissucol in hepatic trauma, Tissucol in splenic trauma, Tissucol in vascular emergencies, fibrin sealant, Tissucol

Abstract

From 1982 to 1985, we have used fibrin sealant (Tissucol) in 15 patients urgently operated on for a ruptured aortic aneurism, in 27 patients with hepatic trauma, and in 32 patients with splenic trauma. The sealant was used in order to prevent intraoperative hemorrhages, to accelerate clotting times and to stop the bleeding at the level of the suture stitches. Tissucol appears to be important mostly in hemostasis to reduce the volume of the oozing in the postoperative days and its use can reduce morbidity and days in hospitalization.

Aortic Aneurysm

Introduction

Aortic aneurysm is one of the most dramatic abdominal vascular diseases with a mortality of 100% if not treated. The patient is submitted to surgery with his or her general and metabolic conditions seriously compromized and is often in shock. For the operation, prosthesis of porous material is used and the patient is heparinized. These plants are often followed by an increased blood loss with an aggravation of the prognosis.

Materials and Methods

From the beginning of 1982 to 1985, we used human fibrin seal (Tissucol) in 15 patients urgently operated on for ruptured aortic aneurysms. The procedure was used to prevent intraoperative hemorrhages, to accelerate clotting times and to stop bleeding at the level of the Dacron prosthesis. We used the classic technique, and the aortic graft of knitted Dacron was treated as follows: 7–10 ml Tissucol seal is produced as described in the instructions and homogeneously applied to the prosthesis 5 min before its grafting. Finally, more seal is applied on the stitches and on the suture line.

Fibrin Sealant in Operative Medicine
Traumatology and Orthopaedics – Vol. 7
Edited by G. Schlag, H. Redl
© Springer-Verlag Berlin Heidelberg 1986

Results and Discussion

The prosthesis treated in this way appeared to be perfectly impermeable; so did the suture, which did not need a further hemostasis.

We noticed no systemic reaction to the fibrin seal or a postoperative defibrination syndrome. The mean volume of blood lost from the prosthesis was 270 ml in the 15 patients not treated with Tissucol (historical cases) compared with 180 ml lost in the postoperative course in those where the substance was used ($P = 0.005$).

The real advantages of using Tissucol are not only the reduction in the volume of oozing and reduction of its time course, but the reduction of morbidity and the days in hospital.

Hepatic Trauma

Introduction

Traumatic lesions of the liver are nowadays still a cause of mortality (15%–20%) [1]; the mortality rises up to 50% when lobectomy becomes necessary [2]. The lesions associated with the hepatic trauma are present in 50%–80% of the cases [3]. The lesions that can be attributed to the liver are:

1. Capsular lacerations and/or of the near tissue
2. Presence of devitalized and/or necrotic parts
3. Lacerations of the intra-hepatic biliary system
4. Vascular injuries of the hilum and/or the suprahepatic veins

Materials and Methods

The most important complications after liver operations for trauma are postoperative hemorrhages, the bilious fistulae and the formation of abscesses; we employed Tissucol in a nonrandomized study (because of the non-comparable lesions) in order to obtain a reduction of the above mentioned complications.

From 1982 to March 1985, we have employed Tissucol sealant on 18 patients with superficial hepatic (capsular) lacerations, on 1 patient subjected to hepatic resection (left hepatectomy) and on 8 patients who had a toilet of necrotic and nonvital hepatic parenchyma and were given partial resections. Tissucol sealant is employed in order to improve hemostasis and to seal bilious ductuli not otherwise suturable but still responsable for important secretions in the postoperative period.

1. The capsular lacerations associated with parenchymal lesions are filled with Tissucol (5–7 ml) and the edges are faced.
2. The necrotic parts are widely removed while the residual cavity is covered with Tissucol and filled with hemostatic sponge; a draining tube is set in the area.
3. A segmental resection appeared essential in a penetrating lesion involving the entire left lobe of the liver; since after both biliary and the largest vessels are tied and sutured, an oozing of the field always persists; thus Tissucol (10 ml) and hemostatic sponges were applied over it; we also applied some stitches and drains as usual.

Results and Discussion

In all patients we obtained a safe and definitive intra- and postoperative hemostasis and we satisfactorily avoided a biliary loss, as measured by the scarce drained material. Tissucol sealant appears to be important mostly in hemostasis, thus in the postoperative period, but not in the complications (metabolic) due to the lesions or the loss of hepatic parenchyma.

Splenic Trauma

Introduction

In 1952, Kind and Schumaker [4] demonstrated a significant relationship between splenectomy and the appearance of sepsis, which was particularly serious and sometimes lethal in children. These data were subsequently fully confirmed [5, 6]. Recently a reexamination of the treatment criteria in cases of traumatic lesions of the spleen became mandatory, also accounting for the new anatomical and functional discoveries on splenic structure [7], as for the new surgical technique and materials and for splenic parenchyma transplantation.

In accord with the Toubukian [8] classification, we can distinguish:
a) subcapsular hematoma,
b) parenchymal laceration, and
c) organ crushing.

Materials and Methods

From the beginning of 1982 to March 1985, 22 splenic capsular lesions and 10 parenchymal lacerations have been treated with Tissucol sealant, while cases of radial lesions and spleen crushing have been submitted to splenectomy.
1. In the case of capsular lesions, simple and/or associated with minimal parenchymal damage, 5 ml Tissucol was applied with a hemostatic sponge.
2. In the case of parenchymal lesions, single, double or polar, the nonvascularized and nonvital tissue was excised and Tisscucol seal (5–7 ml) with hemostatic sponge was applied; the parenchyma was then sutured and the splenic site sutured.

Results and Discussion

The selection of patients made it possible to avoid a second radical operation or later hemorrhages. Moreover, the use of fibrin sealant enabled, according to the new conservative views on splenic surgery, the number of splenectomies to be reduced. The even partial preservation of the organ is followed by a minimal level of morbidity and no mortality at all. Tissucol seal associated with other technical expedients represents for us a valid mean for the conservative treatment of traumatic splenic lesions.

References

1. Defore WW, Mattox KL, Jordan GL, and Beall AC (1976) management of 1 590 consecutive cases of liver trauma Arch Surg 111, 593–597
2. Balesegaram M (1976) The surgical management of hepatic trauma. J of Trauma 16, 141–148
3. Trunkey DD, Shires GT, Mc Celland R (1974) Management of liver trauma in 811 consecutive patients. Ann Surg 179, 722–728
4. King H, Schumaker HB (1952) Susceptibility of infection after splenectomy performed in infancy. Ann Surg 136, 239–242
5. Eraklis AJ, Filler RM (1972) Splenectomy in childhood: a review of 1 413 cases. J of Pediatric Surgery 7, 382–388
6. Dickermann JD (1976) Bacterial infection and the splenic host: a review J of trauma 16, 662–668
7. Esperança Pina JA, Borges D'Almeida J (1980) Anatomo-clinical basis for conservative surgery of the spleen. Abstract Collegium Internationale Chirurgiae Digestivae, II, 10–31 Lisbon
8. Touloukian RJ (1978) Abdominal injuries in Pediatric trauma ed by RJ Touloukian; 377 New York John Willey and Son

III. Orthopaedics

The Effect of the Fibrin Adhesion System on Bone Tissue

P. Bösch, F. Lintner, and G. Kellner

Key words: Bone grafting, experimental investigations

Abstract

A survey is given of the experimental investigations and comparative clinical studies of fibrin-spongiosa grafting performed by the authors over a period of 10 years; their own positive results are critically compared with those reported in other works.

Introduction

The effect of fibrin sealant on bone tissue can only be appraised in comparison with the natural blood clot. The fibrin sealant takes the place of the natural haematoma which fills the interfragment space in fractures, osteotomies or between bone grafts and the osseous bed. The sealant has sufficient strength to anchor osteochondritic fragments in their (exactly fitting) original beds or to clot-weld cancellous bone grafts and fix them in the bone defect. The remodelling of bone grafts is directly dependent on their union with the vascular system. Therefore, early replacement of the fibrin clot by abundantly vascularized granulation tissue is essential to conduce remodelling of the adjacent portions of bone tissue. The fibrin adhesion system is applied to bone tissue chiefly for its capacity to promote the proliferation of new vessels (Table 1).

Table 1. Determinants of biological or biomechanical characteristics of the fibrin adhesion system

Organization of the fibrin seal	versus	Persistence of the fibrin seal
Concentrated fibrinogen		Concentrated fibrinogen
Higher thrombin concentration (600 IU) (rapid polymerization)		Thrombin concentration (can be varied to determine the setting rate)
Factor XIII content		Factor XIII content
Fibronectin content		————
———— (antifibrinolytics inhibit vascularization!)		Addition of antifibrinolytics (aprotinin, EACA)
Use of homologous fibrin sealant		Use of heterologous fibrin sealant

Fibrin Sealant in Operative Medicine
Traumatology and Orthopaedics – Vol. 7
Edited by G. Schlag, H. Redl
© Springer-Verlag Berlin Heidelberg 1986

Material and Method

All the materials and methods used in the course of our studies have been described in detail in earlier papers by the authors.

Results

Survey of Experimental Investigations Made by the Authors

We started our investigations of the fibrin sealant system in bone tissue by studying the healing process of bore holes drilled into rabbit tibiae. When the defects were filled with *human* fibrin sealant bone healing was completely suppressed in the first 2 weeks. Thereafter, the fibrin sealant was gradually replaced by callus. During the 5-week observation period only partial healing occurred. When homologous fibrin sealant was used, defect healing was somewhat faster than in the control group. In numerous subsequent experiments we invariably used homologous fibrin sealant without adding aprotinin or any other antifibrinolytic substance. Animals in which no sealant was used served as controls. The experimental setting was such as to largely eliminate the factor of additional stabilization exerted by the sealant.

The healing and complete remodelling of autologous bone grafts implanted into the iliac bones of rabbits was accelerated due to the effects of the fibrin sealant, the final results being the same in the test group and in the controls.

The use of the fibrin sealant even led to osseous incorporation of heterologous, cancellous Kiel bone grafts, whose trabeculae were surrounded by new bone prior to secondary osteoblastic absorption. In the control group, just connective tissue development and osteoclastic breakdown of the implants was seen in all cases after 8 – 12 weeks. The advancing growth of the site spongiosa led to a gradual reduction in size and to increasing ossification of the defect.

The fixation of porous metal cylinders in rabbit tibia is significantly improved and, according to histological evidence, also accelerated.

It was demonstrated that the breaking strength of a double osteotomy, as measured after 5 and 7 weeks, was higher when the sealant was used and the remodelling of the interfragment spaces was more advanced, histologically.

In none of the test groups were remains of the fibrin sealant found at the site of sealing after 1 week, when test animals that happened to die were examined.

Hygienists were able to show that an antibiotic added to the fibrin sealant (clot produced in the medullary space of the rabbit femur) was effective for twice as long as in a comparable antibiotic-blood clot. In vitro, the bacterial growth was significantly greater in the blood clot than in the fibrin seal.

Comparative Clinical Studies Performed by the Authors

The comparative clinical studies of cancellous bone grafting with and without fibrin sealant, performed since 1975, showed that the remodelling of spongiosa implants is distinctly improved by the use of fibrin sealant. This improvement is especially noticeable when heterologous spongiosa grafts are used, but also with homologous bone grafts. The excellent results achieved in osteomyelitic defects by fibrin-spongiosa grafting using heterologous bone is likewise impressive.

Discussion

The experimental studies performed on various animal models indicated that by the use of the fibrin adhesion system the incorporation and remodelling of cancellous bone implants can be clearly improved. The lower the osteoinductive capacity of the cancellous bone grafts, the more distinctive is this effect. Invariably, good results were only obtained when homologous fibrin sealant was used and neither aprotinin nor ε-aminocaproic acid (EACA) was added. The fibrin network of the sealant serves as a conducting medium for ingrowing blood vessels and is replaced by abundantly vascularized granulation tissue within a week. Our comparative clinical studies, performed after exactly 10 years, have clearly confirmed this positive effect of the sealant on the incorporation and remodelling of transplanted bone. When surveying the literature of recent years or the papers presented during this symposium, it is remarkable that no other comparative clinical studies have been performed as yet.

In nearly all of the numerous experimental studies undertaken by other investigators either heterologous fibrin sealant was used or homologous sealant *plus* aprotinin or EACA. Again and again it has been demonstrated histologically that remains of the sealant persist even after several weeks, though we have never been able to make this finding. This is somewhat perplexing, because we pointed out this obvious source of error in our first papers on the subject published in 1977. The fibrin sealant should just serve as a conductive medium for the proliferation of granulation tissue. Moreover, vascularization is promoted by the mechanical stabilization due to the sealant. The addition of antifibrinolytics, which is certainly necessary in operations on the urogenital tract or in other fields of surgery, prevents early vascular union. If the sealant layers are very thin, as in the fixation of osteochondral fragments, the mechanical strength may be in the foreground and the inhibiting effect exerted by the "fibrin sealant system inducing antifibrinolytics" may not be overly pronounced.

Our controlled, comparative clinical studies performed over a period of about 10 years corroborate the merits of fibrin-spongiosa grafting, especially in large, in osteomyelitic, and in haemophilic defects and when using bone grafts other than autologous spongiosa.

References

Bösch P (1981) Die Fibrinspongiosaplastik. Wien klin Wschr 93, Suppl 124

Clinical Experiences with the Use of the Fibrin-Antibiotic Complex Nebacetin in the Treatment of Chronic Bone Infections and as a Prophylactic Against Infections in Cases of Non-infected Bone and Soft Tissue Defects

Y.M. GOUDARZI

Key words: Clinical experiences with the fibrin-antibiotic complex

Abstract

In view of our experiences, the use of the fibrin-antibiotic complex (Nebacetin) opens new possibilities in the supplementary local treatment of bone and soft tissue infections. When using fibrin as a physiological carrier substance, highly concentrated doses of Nebacetin are released at the site of the infection. Fibrin has the advantages of good malleability and of an optimal coagulative property, which helps prevent hematomas in the wound area. Fibrin-antibiotic complex in combination with synthetic skin is well suited to the temporary covering of open wounds, especially after compound fractures and defects of the skin and soft tissue. It protects the wound against bacterial invasion and stimulates the granulation of the wound, until definitive closure by means of autogenous skin graft or delayed suture. The use of this treatment can achieve a significant reduction of osteitis and infection. Since 1979, we have treated 44 children with the fibrin-antibiotic complex. Autologous bone grafting was carried out on 37 patients. Furthermore, we treated seven cases with compound fractures and extensive soft tissue damage without involvement of the bone. Nebacetin provides a most effective local antibiotic therapy as supplementary and consecutive treatment after surgical procedures executed in bone infections. The chronic bone infections of 19 children subsided completely. In 18 children with bone transplants, no infection was observed and all the patients showed primary healing. After 12 weeks, the establishment of normal bone structure was almost complete. In only two cases did we have to operate again, due to recurrent bone cysts. In seven cases with compound fractures and extensive soft tissue damage, we were able to prevent infection. Two weeks later an ideal base for autodermic grafting or delayed suture was attained. We observed no hepatitis in our patients. The surgical technique and advantages of treatment are discussed.

Introduction

Even in the age of antibiotics, the medical treatment of chronic bone infections, with their various courses and unpredictable recurrences, is a surgical problem.

When treating a chronic bone infection, the local therapy measures, as well as the surgical removal of necrosis of the soft tissue and of the bones, the creation of

Fibrin Sealant in Operative Medicine
Traumatology and Orthopaedics – Vol. 7
Edited by G. Schlag, H. Redl
© Springer-Verlag Berlin Heidelberg 1986

sufficient stability, and the refilling of bone defects with autologous spongiosa are of crucial importance.

Through the increasing failure of systemic antibiotic therapy, local antibacterial chemotherapy used as a supplement to surgical treatment of bone and soft tissue infections has gained in clinical importance.

The successful use of bone cements [3] consisting of antibiotics and gentamycin-PMMA chains (PMMA, polymethylmethacrylate) [6], brought the knowledge that the implantation of antibiotic carriers, directly at the site of the infection, allows for the achievement of optimum levels of antibiotic concentration. The disadvantage of the PMMA chains is that polymethylmethacrylate is a foreign body substance that must be combined with further narcosis in order to be removed 10–14 days later. The use of a fibrin polymerizate as a physiological carrier substance for antibiotics in animal experiments on the treatment of bone and soft tissue infections resulted in favorable reports [1, 2]. The conclusions gained from these animal experiments have, in the mean time, been clinically confirmed several times [5, 7]. Since 1979, in therapy as well as in the prophylaxis of the autologous osteoplastic refilling of bone defects, osteomyelitical foci, and soft tissue defects, we have been applying fibrin with an admixture of Nebacetin.

Material and Method

To date (February 1985), 44 children have been treated with the fibrin-Nebacetin complex in the Pediatric Surgical Department of the Rudolf-Virchow Hospital in Berlin. Indications for the use of the compound were osteomyelitis 19 times, noninfected bone defects 18 times, compound lower leg fractures twice and extensive soft tissue defects five times. Gender of patient, average age, location of affection, and type of affection are shown in Table 1.

For the construction of the fibrin-Nebacetin complex, 2 ml human fibrinogen (Tissucol) with 32 500 IU (50 mg) Neomycinsulfate and 2500 IU baciteracin in siccum form are mixed, and through the addition of 1 ml thrombin are brought to polymerization. Hereby, a gel-like substance is created, which is then mixed with the autologous spongiosa. In the bone part which is to be refilled, *debridement* of the soft tissue and sequesterotomy are carried out. Immediately afterwards, the healthy bone marrow is opened.

For the supply of blood to the implanted spongiosa, the construction of a link to the healthy marrow is of the greatest importance [4, 8]. The bone defect is filled, layerwise, with the fibrin-Nebacetin-spongiosa mixture. After the attachment of an overflow drain, the wound is closed off, layerwise.

In the treatment of soft tissue defects, the removal of necrosis is followed by a temporary wound dressing of the fibrin-Nebacetin complex and the synthetic skin substitute Geliperm to prevent infections until definitive wound closure is accomplished by means of secondary suture or plastic measures. Before the application of the fibrin-Nebacetin complex, the pathogenic organism was identified and its sensitivity to Nebacetin was determined by the antibiogram. Kidney and liver functions were scrutinized before and after surgery.

Table 1. Surgical treatment of bone and soft tissue infections with fibrin-antibiotic-compound in the Pediatric Surgical Department of the Rudolf-Virchow Hospital, Berlin (current: February 1985)

Number of patients	44
Male	28
Female	16
Average age	11 years 4 months
Diagnose	
Juvenile bone cysts	15
Thereof pathological fractures	(8)
Non infected pseudarthroses	3
Chronic osteomyelitis	19
Thereof infected osteosyntheses	(3)
Compound lower leg fractures with soft tissue problems	2
Extensive soft tissue defects	5
Localization of the chronic osteomyelitis	
Upper extremity, shoulder girdle, shoulder joint, and upper arm	3
Elbow joint	2
Lower arm and hand	4
Lower extremity, pelvis, hip joint	3
Thigh	2
Lower leg, ankle, and foot	5

The following are examples of the clinical usage:

K. J.: Seven-year-old girl with severe chronic osteomyelitis with fistula of the radius. The fistula smear shows *Staphylococcus aureus,* which is sensitive to Nebacetin, to be the pathogenic organism. Surgical revision and filling with fibrin-Nebacetin complex and autologous spongiosa. Primary wound healing, and after 4 months, complete reconstruction of the spongiosa without bone scarring and absence of recurrence.

T. O.: Thirteen-year-old boy. Chronic osteomyelitis in the left calcaneus in a state after hematogenous osteomyelitis. Pathogenic organism: *Staphylococcus aureus.* Surgical revision and treatment with fibrin-Nebacetin and autologous spongiosa. Primary wound healing, subsidence of infection, and absence of recurrences (Figs. 1, 2).

E. O.: Thirteen-year-old boy with post-traumatic osteomyelitis after surgical treatment of a proximal fracture of the right ulna. Surgical revision, sequesterotomy, and filling with fibrin-Nebacetin complex. Primary wound healing and subsidence of infection.

J. D.: Thirteen-year-old girl with extensive circular skin and soft tissue necrosis in the area of the left lower leg. Pathogenic organism: *Staphylococcus aureus, Enterococci,* and *hemolytic streptococci* Group A. Necrosis removal and temporary covering with fibrin-Nebacetin complex and Geliperm. Dressing changed every 2 days. After 10 days, there is definitive wound closure through skin grafts (Figs. 3, 4).

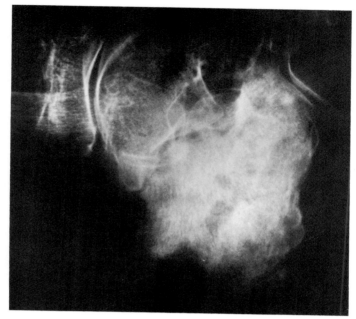

Fig. 1. Chronic osteomyelitis of the left os calsis

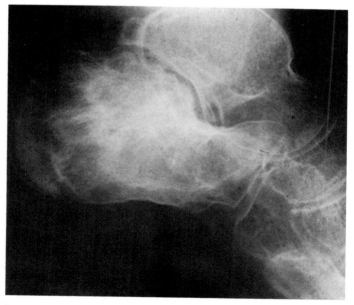

Fig. 2. Primary healing after surgical revision and refilling with fibrin-Nebacetin compound

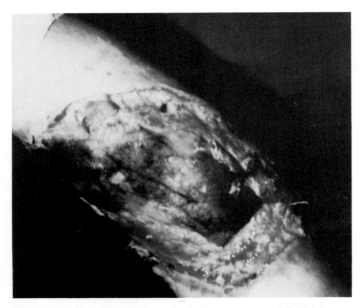

Fig. 3. Extensive circular skin and soft tissue necroses of the left lower leg

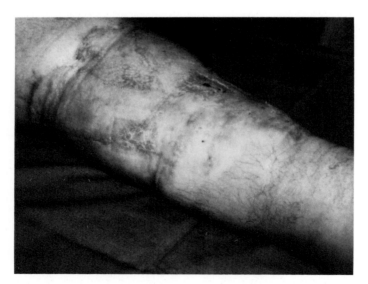

Fig. 4. Condition after skin transplantation following removal of necroses and temporary covering with fibrin-Nebacetin compound

J. K.: Seven-year-old polytraumatic girl with traumatic amputation of the left lower leg, with massive contusions and severe destruction of the soft tissue cover, including the destruction of the underlying muscles, blood vessels, nerves, and bones. The severity of the contusions and lacerations unfortunately did not allow for a replantation attempt. Our endeavors had to aim at saving the functionally extremely important knee joint. During the postoperative period, extensive necrosis developed in the area of the stump of the lower leg. After the removal of the necrosis, we temporarily covered the wound with fibrin-Nebacetin complex and the synthetic skin substitute Geliperm. The bandage was renewed every 2 days, and after 10 days we were able to cover the stump with skin grafts.

Results

After the implantation of fibrin-Nebacetin complex with autologous spongiosa in noninflammatory bone foci, no postoperative infections were registered. The bone implantation and reconstruction processes were not hampered by the use of fibrin cements. The bony connection of the autologous spongiosa in the transplantation area was completed by the 12th postoperative week. The results are shown in Table 2. Two recurrent cysts came into observation after the primary operation. In 19 children with a chronic bone infection, subsidence of infection and primary wound healing were achieved. In the cases of two compound fractures and in five cases of extensive soft tissue defects, infection was prevented until wound closure by way of secondary suture, i.e., skin transplantation could be achieved. No hepatitis was observed in our patients.

Table 2. Surgical treatment of bone and soft tissue infections with fibrin-antibiotic-compound in the Pediatric Surgical Department of the Rudolf-Virchow Hospital, Berlin (current: February 1985) ($n = 44$)

Juvenile bone cysts	15
Thereof primary wound healing	(15)
Thereof recurrent cysts	(2)
Non infected pseudarthroses	3
Thereof primary wound healing	(3)
Chronic osteomyelitis	19
Primary wound healing and subsidence of infection	(19)
Compound fractures with soft tissue problems and extensive soft tissue defects without bone involvement	7
Prevention of infection until definitive closure of wound by way of secondary suture or plastic methods	(7)

References

1. Braun A, Schumacher G, Kratzat R, Heine WD, Pasch B (1981) Der Fibrin-Antibioticum-Verbund im Tierexperiment zur lokalen Therapie des staphylokokkeninfizierten Knochens. Heft zur Unfallheilkunde 148: 809-811

2. Braun A, Schumacher G, Kratzat R, Heine WD, Pasch B, Fabricius K (1981) Der Fibrin-Antibiotikum-Verbund im Tierexperiment, Heft zur Unfallheilkunde, 153: 83-86
3. Buchholz, HW, Engelbrecht H (1970) Über Depotwirkung einiger Antibiotica bei Vermischung mit Kunstharz (Palaeos). Chirurg 40: 511.
4. Demmler K (1976) Das Gefäßsystem des Knochenmarks (Bücherei des Orthopäden Vol. 15) Stuttgart – F Enke
5. Goudarzi Y M (1983)Klinische Erfahrungen mit einer Fibrin-Nebacetin-Spongiosaplombe zur Behandlung der chronischen Knocheninfektionen und als lokale Infektionsprophylaxe bei nicht infiziertem Knochenherd. Akt Traumatol 13: 205-209.
6. Klemm K (1977) Gentamycin-PMMA-Ketten, eine Alternative zu Spül-Saug-Drainagen bei Knochen- und Weichteilinfektionen. Langenbeck Arch Chir 345: 609.
7. Kratzat R, Braun A, Schumacher G (1982) Klinische Erfahrungen mit Fibrin-Antibioticum-Verbund bei Knochen- und Weichteilinfektionen. Akt Chir No 2 Vol 17.
8. Sauer K, ambe LT, Schweiberer L (1978)Experimentelle Untersuchungen zum Einbau autologer Spongiosa in die Kompakta des Röhrenknochens. Arch ortho Traumat Surg 92: 211

Preparation and Application of Fibrin-antibiotic Complex

A. Braun

Key words: Fibrin-antibiotic complex, spongiosa transplantations, bone and soft tissue infections

Abstract

As supplementary local treatment in bone and soft tissue infections and in spongiosa transplantations endangered by infection, fibrin-antibiotic complex serves as prophylactic therapy, since the not yet vascularized spongiosa transplant is poorly accessible to a systemic antibiotic treatment. The advantage of exogenous human fibrin as the carrier substance of the antibiotic is that this physiological matrix is eliminated under the action of local fibrinolysis. Experimental, clinical as well as pharmacokinetic investigations and results have shown that the fibrin-antibiotic complex affords appreciable clinical advantages [1–18, 10–12, 14–18]. We use almost exclusively gentamicin sulfate as antibiotic. Since we frequently mix isogeneic or allogeneic spongiosa with the fibrin-gentamicin complex, and also fill sinuses with this complex, its preparation and the technique of application will be described below.

Fibrin-gentamicin complex in bone and soft tissue infections

In acute and chronic infections of bone and soft tissue, fibrin-gentamicin complex is only an adjuvant local therapy. Surgical debridement and immobilization have therapeutic priority. Alloplastic implants and sequesters must be removed, and necrotic bone and soft tissue must be resected. If it is not removed, eburnated and sclerotic bone should if possible be drilled in order to obtain connection with vascularized tissue. The osteomyelitic cavity carefully curetted with a spherical cutter is filled with fibrin-gentamicin complex. When there is a poor bone bed, large defects and if inadequate osteoneosynthesis is to be expected, we use the fibrin-gentamicin-spongiosa complex exclusively. In all cases, an antibiogram should be available, and the sensitivity of the bacteria to gentamicin should have been tested. Creatinine and urea values should be in the normal range in order to ensure excretion of eluted gentamicin in the urine.

In small bone defects in which good osseous consolidation is to be expected without additional spongiosa transplantation, we occasionally still use fibrin-gentamicin complex. We have also used fibrin-gentamicin complex without spongiosa reconstruction after surgical debridement and immobilization in bacterial infections on the sternoclavicular joint as well as on the symphysis. After surgical preparation

Fibrin Sealant in Operative Medicine
Traumatology and Orthopaedics – Vol. 7
Edited by G. Schlag, H. Redl
© Springer-Verlag Berlin Heidelberg 1986

of the cavity to be filled, the total amount of complex required must be estimated. If appraisal is difficult, a 10 ml syringe with Ringer solution can be helpful in determining the volume. The fibrin-gentamicin complex consists of three components and is mixed extracorporeally in a small metal or ceramic dish until the initial crosslinking occurs. 50% of the required total amount should consist of highly concentrated human fibrin (Tissucol/Tisseel) for which we use the deep-frozen commercially available form in the thawed state. The antibiotic is added as second component to fibrinogen. To prepare the antibiotic solution, 500 mg gentamicin sulfate in powder form is dissolved with 1 ml distilled water. If a large total amount of complex is required, 2 ml distilled water can also be used. Commercially available Refobacin in a quantity of 40 or 80 mg gentamicin is dissolved in 1 or 2 ml respectively, so that the amount of gentamicin activity is reduced in practical application (especially in small bone cavities) that in comparative terms only a low-dose local antibiotic therapy is possible. In patients over 50 kg body weight, 500 mg gentamicin sulfate can be used when kidney function is intact. A high gentamicin activity is thus present in a volume unit of 1 ml. In patients with a lower body weight, about 10 mg gentamicin per kg body weight must be calculated. Pharmacokinetic investigations [6] have shown that the serum and urinary levels of gentamicin resulting from 10 mg per kg body weight after application in fibrin complex do not exceed the serum and urinary levels resulting from 80 mg Refobacin administered i.m. In addition, loss of gentamicin is to be expected owing to biological inactivation of aminoglycoside, as well as a loss in wound secretion and in the drainage system [6]. In mixing small amounts (1–2 ml) of fibrinogen and highly concentrated gentamicin solution (500 mg/ml), premature clotting may occasionally occur. However, in our experience this does not have any disadvantageous effect on the complex. As a third component, a solution containing thrombin is used in order to crosslink fibrinogen to fibrin. Since the elution rate of the antibiotic does not depend on the elimination rate of the fibrin clot, we dispense with the use of fibrinolysis inhibitors. Since the rate of coagulation of the fibrinogen-gentamicin mixture in the fibrin-gentamicin complex is delayed by about two minutes by the antibiotic [12], we use the high thrombin concentration (bottle "D" from the application set for deepfrozen fibrin tissue adhesive sealant). From bottle "B", 3 ml (0.5 or 1 ml application set) or 6 ml (2 ml application set) calcium chloride solution in bottle "D" with 500 IU thrombin (0.5 or 1 ml application set) or 1000 IU thrombin (2 ml application set) is transferred and the thrombin is dissolved. The extracorporeal preclotting of the complex is commenced by admixture of the solution containing thrombin. For this purpose, 50% of the total complex is required analogous to the amount of fibrin or 50% minus the amount of gentamicin solution. After careful mixing with a Kocher trough, the complex is filled into the nonbleeding bone cavity with visible coagulation (after about two minutes). If possible, the soft tissue mantle should be primarily closed. As drainage, we use a small silicone tube for 24 hours without suction. We have not observed major secretion.

	Rule of thumb: fibrin-gentamicin complex
A	50% human fibrinogen (Tissucol/Tisseel)
B	gentamicin sulfate (10 mg/kg body weight – maximum 500 mg) in 1 ml distilled water
C	50% high-concentration thrombin solution (application set "B" in "D") minus 1 ml (= amount of gentamicin sulfate solution)

A + B + (C–B) = total amount

e.g.   A ⟶ 4 ml Tissucol/Tisseel
              B ⟶ 1 ml gentamicin sulfate solution
     (C–B) ⟶ 3 ml (4 ml – 1 ml) solution containing thrombin

Total amount: 8 ml fibrin-gentamicin complex

Fibrin-gentamicin-spongiosa complex

Although we have seen good osteoneosynthesis in numerous cases when using the fibrin-gentamicin complex alone [7], osteoneosynthesis had not occurred in occasional cases. We therefore decided to apply a fibrin-gentamicin-spongiosa complex in almost all cases of a bone defect in osteomyelitis or osteitis in past years. Since a poor bone bed ist almost always present in infections, exclusively isogeneic spongiosa should be used. The spongiosa is always removed before the septic operation in the same session, if possible from the dorsal iliac crest. Both surgical areas are exposed separately. So far, we have not observed an infection on the iliac crest. The isogeneic spongiosa is stored in isogeneic blood from the wound until further processing is carried out.

The bone cavity or the bone defect is prepared as described above. The fibrin-gentamicin-spongiosa complex consists of four components and is likewise mixed extracorporeally in a small metal or ceramic dish until the initial crosslinking commences. So far, there have been no experimental investigations as to the relation of isogeneic spongiosa and fibrin-gentamicin complex which provides the optimal precondition for osteoneosynthesis. On the basis of clinical experience, we prefer a relation of spongiosa to fibrin-gentamicin complex of 5–10:1. A precise establishment of the quantitative relation is difficult owing to individual circumstances. In practical application, it is proved to be advantageous to use sufficient spongiosa to fill the bone defect without compression of the spongiosa. Large spongiosa fragments should be chopped up with the Liston to roughly the size of lentils or beans.

As described on page 171, a mixture of highly concentrated human fibrinogen (Tissucol/Tisseel) and gentamicin sulfate solution is prepared (Fig. 1). Depending on the size of the defect to be filled, 0.5–8 ml of commercially available fibrinogen

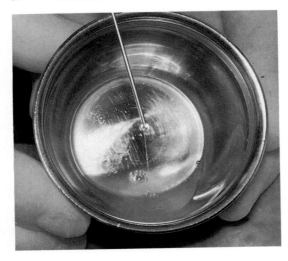

Fig. 1. Mixture of fibrinogen and gentamicin sulfate solution

(Tissucol/Tisseel) is required. In most cases in our clinical study [7, 8], between 2 and 4 ml were required. The amount of gentamicin depends on the body weight (cf. page 173). The chopped spongiosa is added to the mixture of fibrinogen and gentamicin sulfate and mixed until the entire surface of the spongiosa is coated with fibrin-gentamicin (Fig. 2). The gentamicin-enriched fibrinogen adheres to the bone so well that it is hardly visible any longer. The solution containing thrombin is now added as described above and the complex is placed in the tamponaded bone defect during the transformation of fibrinogen to fibrin. The spongiosa is slightly compressed with the fingertip or with a pestle. After about five minutes, most of the fibrin has been crosslinked. It is astonishing how the modelled spongiosa is held in the fibrin complex, e.g. in bridging over defects in the bone. If possible, the wound is

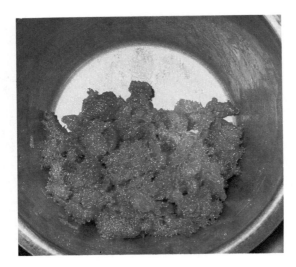

Fig. 2. Autologous spongiosa surface-coated with fibrin-gentamicin complex

closed primarily. Special importance is to be attached to immobilization. The duration of immobilization depends on whether there is a severance of the bone continuity. In about 50% of our cases, we have administered a systemic antibiotic in addition. Care should be taken that it acts synergistically with gentamicin.

A progress observation after use of fibrin-gentamicin-spongiosa complex in a defect infection pseudarthrosis of the ulna is shown as an example. The ulna is shown preferentially here, because pseudarthrosis of the ulna constitutes a substantial problem of therapy.

The 21 year old female patient suffered a third-degree compound fracture of the left forearm. The ulna and radius were treated with a plate osteosynthesis. There was early infection. In surgical revision, gentamicin-PMMA beads were inserted (Fig. 3a). The infection on the radius was suppressed. In persistent infection on the ulnar side, the plate of the ulna was removed and a fixateur externe was applied (Fig. 3b). By application of the fibrin-antibiotic complex, *a single-session procedure* was possible. After removal of fresh isogeneic spongiosa from the iliac crest, a local debridement was carried out (Fig. 3c). Fixateur externe, gentamicin-PMMA beads, sequester and screws were removed, and the avital bone ends were trimmed. The

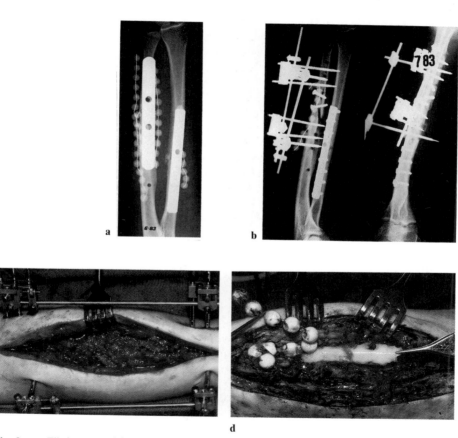

Fig. 3 a–g. Fibrin-gentamicin-spongiosa complex in a defect infection pseudarthrosis of the ulna

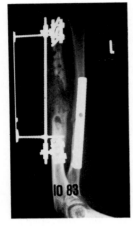
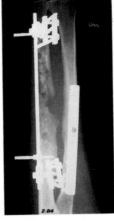

Fig. 3 e   Fig. 3 f

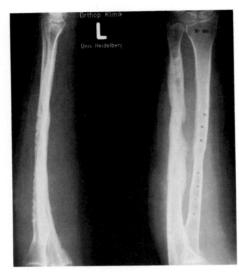

Fig. 3 g

ulna was immobilized by reapplication of a fixateur externe. The defect was filled with fibrin-gentamicin-spongiosa complex (Fig. 3d and e). Primary skin closure is possible. There was no recurrence of the infection. Increasing bone union (Fig. 3f) up to complete bony bridging (Fig. 3g).

The example shows that debridement and immobilization constitute fundamental preconditions for suppression of infections and that spongiosa grafting promotes bone healing. The antibiotic in the fibrin complex serves as an important local adjuvant therapy.

In 1985 [8], we reported the first time on a cement-free prosthesis implantation at the knee joint with fibrin-gentamicin-spongiosa complex. The infected endoprosthesis was removed with the loosened cement complex. With gentamicin-PMMA beads (Septopal), primary wound closure and immobilization in fixateur externe, the infection could be brought under control. Isogeneic and allogeneic spongiosa with fibrin-gentamicin complex was used for cement-free prosthetic reimplantation (Fig. 6f). A very substantial amount of bone substance could thus be obtained with sustained suppression of the infection.

Rule of thumb: fibrin-gentamicin-spongiosa complex	
I	fibrin-gentamicin complex
II	isogenic (allogeneic) spongiosa
I:II = 1:(5 to 10)	
Fibrin-gentamicin-spongiosa complex (I) preparation: – mix human fibrinogen (Tissucol/Tisseel) – in gentamicin sulfate solution (10 mg gentamicin sulfate per kg body weight – maximum 500 mg – in 1–2 ml distilled water – use mixture for surface coating of isogeneic (allogeneic) spongiosa (II) – before application add highly concentrated thrombin solution (application set "B" in "D") minus the amount of gentamicin sulfate (= 1 ml)	
I + II = total amount I = A + B (C–B) analogous to the rule of thumb on page 173	

Fibrin-gentamicin complex for filling sinuses

It is inconsistent with the principle of treatment in septic surgery to close an infected sinus without clearing the source of the sinus. Nevertheless, spontaneous closures of an infected sinus have been described after contrast medium imaging [9, 13]. The idea that the sinus can be sealed by the fibrin-gentamicin complex, formation of granulation tissue is promoted and a bactericidal antibiotic concentration is applied in the sinus has caused us to fill sinuses under certain conditions. Metallic implants, sequesters and non-resorbable suture material associated with the sinus are contraindications. So far, sinus glueing was only carried out in patients in whom a surgical revision of the sinus entailed substantial risks. We have been applying the method since 1981 and could suppress the infection in about half of all the more than 50 cases. The bacterium should be sensitive to gentamicin and the creatinine and urea values should be in the normal range.

We estimate the amount of fibrin-gentamicin complex required after prior sinography (Fig. 4). If the estimated total volume of the sinus is less than 4 ml, we use the double syringe from the application set for deep-frozen Tissucol/Tisseel fibrin tissue adhesive sealant (2 ml) for injection. If the sinus volume is more than 4 ml, we mix the fibrin-gentamicin complex in a 20 ml disposable syringe.

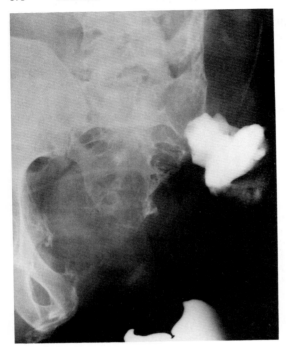

Fig. 4. Contrast imaging of the sinus. 32 year old patient, traumatic hemipelvectomy on the left. Multiple scar correction, persistent sinus. Estimation of the volume required by contrast imaging. Spontaneous closure after filling with fibrin-gentamicin complex and compression dressing

Application with double syringe of a total volume of up to 4 ml

On the one side of the double syringe, there is 2 ml thawed fibrinogen (Tissucol/Tisseel). On the other side, 1 ml gentamicin sulfate (cf. page 171) is drawn into a 2 ml syringe and its volume increased to 2 ml with a solution containing thrombin (Fig. 5a). The solution containing thrombin is prepared as described on page 173. 1000 IU thrombin from the application set for 2 ml deep-frozen Tissucol/Tisseel fibrin tissue adhesive sealant (bottle "D") are dissolved in 6 ml calcium chloride solution (bottle "B") and 1 ml of this is used. Since the complex must have a high initial flow capacity in order to fill the sinus system, it is not advisable that the thrombin concentration is too high. Using a bulbous cannula, the content of both syringes is injected simultaneously into the sinus with the double syringe. The sinus

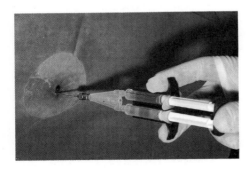

Fig. 5a. In a sinus of up to 4 ml volume, the double syringe was used. The solution containing fibrinogen, gentamicin and thrombin is only mixed in the sinus system

opening is compressed with a compress during injection and for about five minutes afterwards. The bulbous cannula should be rinsed immediately after injection in order to avoid fibrin clots in the cannula.

Application of a total volume of more than 4 ml with a disposable syringe

50% of the total amount of the complex of thawed brinelike fibrinogen (Tissucol/ Tisseel) is drawn up into a 20 ml disposable syringe (Fig. 5b). A solution containing thrombin which should also contain 1 ml gentamicin sulfate depending on the body weight (for concentration, cf. page 173) are added to 50% of the total amount of the complex. We prefer the low-concentration thrombin solution in which 4 IU thrombin from the application set for 2 ml deep-frozen Tissucol/Tisseel fibrin tissue adhesive sealant (bottle "C") are dissolved with 3 ml calcium chloride (bottle "D"). The low thrombin concentration is important so that extensive consolidation which would prevent injection via the bulbous cannula into the sinus does not already occur in the syringe. The injection should be carried out quickly. The sinus opening is compressed during injection and for about five minutes afterwards. Rinse bulbous cannula immediately after use!

After each filling of a sinus with fibrin-gentamicin complex, a compression bandage should be applied. The sinus can then close spontaneously. Good results were still obtained when a slight secretion was observed from the sinus over a few days. In two cases in which the bacterium was not sensitive to gentamicin, the sinus was filled with fibrin-cefotaxim complex.

Fibrin-gentamicin complex in spongiosa graft endangered by infection

Although allogenic spongiosa stored by deep-freezing is not comparable with isogeneic spongiosa in its osteogenetic potency, we have obtained good results in filling large bone cavities, especially in children and adolescents. The allogeneic bone is removed intraoperatively in head and neck resections of the hip joint or from cadavers within the first six hours after death. It is implanted after being stored deep-frozen in the bone bank. Although removal and storage are sterile, there is danger of contamination. Since the implanted allogeneic bone is avital until it is

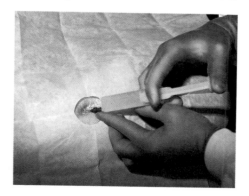

Fig. 5b. In a sinus of over 4 ml volume, a 20 ml syringe is used. After mixing fibrinogen, gentamicin and thrombin solution in the syringe, immediate application is necessary

converted into lamellar bone, there is danger of infection which has poor accessibility to system antibiotic prophylaxis in the absent vascularization of the implanted bone. Here, fibrin-gentamicin complex implanted with the allogeneic bone appears to be more logical, apart from the more favorable conditions of healing induced by the fibrin, as described by Bösch et al. (1977). The fibrin-gentamicin complex may also constitute a supplementary local antibiotic treatment in open fractures requiring spongiosa grafting.

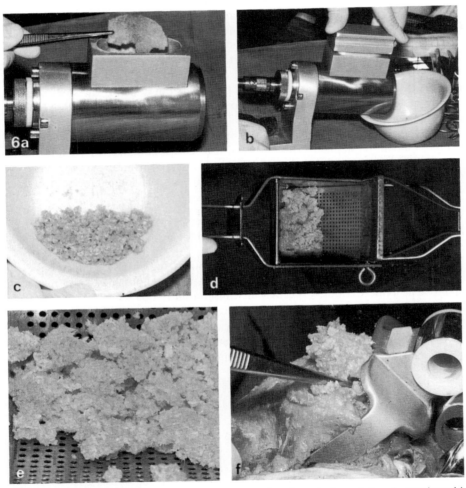

Fig. 6 a–f. *a* A deep-frozen cancellous or corticocancellous bone is thawed; *b* and comminuted in the bone mill; *c* The bone is collected in a dish and washed with warm Ringer solution; *d* and freed mechanically from medullary fat in a hand press; *e* The allogeneic bone substance can be used in this form; *f* The bone substance is used for implantation with the fibrin-gentamicin complex (e.g. cement-free prosthetic reimplantation on the knee joint)

Most bone preparations deep-frozen in corticocancellous blocks are thawed at room temperature and comminuted into coarse bone meal with a bone mill (Aesculap, Tuttlingen) (Fig. 6a–c). By washing several times with Ringer solution at about 60° C and compression by a kind of "potato press" (Fig. 6d–f), the medullary fat which is not required can be largely removed, so that mainly bone substance can be employed for transplantation. The bone substance left behind can be mixed with isogeneic spongiosa. The further processing to fibrin-gentamicin-spongiosa complex is carried out as described on page 173.

The readily formable fibrin-gentamicin-spongiosa complex can be used in many ways during the transformation of fibrinogen to fibrin. Besides application in large bone defects and marginally curetted tumors, spongiosa grafts can be carried out in revision surgery of the acetabular component and in the shaft in cement-free prosthetic implants.

References

1. Bösch P, Braun F, Spängler HP (1977) Die Technik der Fibrin-Spongiosaplastik. Arch Orthop Unfall Chir 90: 63
2. Braun A, Kratzat R, Heine WD, Pasch B (1980) Der Fibrin-Antibiotikum-Verbund im Tierexperiment zur lokalen Therapie des staphylokokkeninfizierten Knochens. Hefte Unfall-heilk 148: 809
3. Braun A, Schumacher G, Kratzat R, Heine WD, Pasch B (1982) Erste klinische Erfahrungen mit dem Fibrin-Tobramycin-Verbund bei Knocheninfektionen. Hefte Unfallheilk 157: 66
4. Braun A, Wahlig H, Dingeldein E (1982) Freisetzungskinetik von Gentamycin nach klinischer Anwendung des Fibrin-Gentamycin-Verbundes bei der Osteomyelitis. Vortrag: 69. Tagung der Deutschen Gesellschaft für Orthopädie und Traumatologie, Mainz
5. Braun A, Schumacher G, Kratzat R, Heine WD, Pasch B, Roesler H (1982) Der Fibrin-Antibiotikum-Verbund im Tierexperiment. In Cotta H, Braun A (Hrsg) Fibrinkleber in Orthopädie und Traumatologie, Thieme, Stuttgart 172–177
6. Braun A, Güssbacher A, Wahlig H, Dingeldein E (1984) Der Fibrin-Antibiotikum-Verbund als ergänzende Lokalbehandlung der Osteomyelitis. In: Scheele J (Hrsg) Fibrinklebung. Springer, Heidelberg 205–210
7. Braun A, Güssbacher A, Heine WD, Dingeldein E (1985) Fibrin-Antibiotic-Complex: Laborat-ory Investigation and Clinical Results. In: Uhthoff H (Hrsg) Current Concepts of Infections in Orthopaedic Surgery. Springer, Heidelberg 265–294
8. Braun A, Lücke R, Ewerbeck V, Dingeldein E Der Fibrin-Gentamicin-Verbund in Orthopädie und Traumatologie Vortrag: Symposium Knochen- und Gelenkinfektionen – Diagnose und Therapie, Heidelberg 13. und 14. September, in press
9. Egkher E, Spängler H (1982) Zum Phänomen des Spontanverschlusses von osteomyelitischen Fisteln nach Kontrastmittelfüllungen. In: Poigenfürst J (Hrsg) Hefte zur Unfallheilk, 157, Springer, Heidelberg 277–281
10. Goudarzi YM (1983) Klinische Erfahrungen mit einer Fibrin-Nebacetin-Spongiosaplombe zur Behandlung der chronischen Knocheninfektion und als lokale Infektionsprophylaxe bei nicht infizierten Knochenherden. Akt Traumatol 13: 205
11. Kratzat R, Braun A, Schumacher G (1982) Erste klinische Erfahrungen mit dem Fibrin-Antibiotikum-Verbund bei Knochen- und Weichteilinfektionen. Akt Chir 17: 58
12. Redl H, Stanek G, Hirschl A, Schlag G (1982) Fibrinkleber-Antibiotika-Gemische. Festigkeit und Elutionsverhalten. In: Cotta H, Braun A (Hrsg) Fibrinkleber in Orthopädie und Traumatologie. Thieme, Stuttgart 178–181
13. Rosemeyer B (1973) Beobachtungen über Spontanverschlüsse von Fisteln nach Kontrastdar-stellung. Arch Othop Unfall Chir 76: 242

182   A. Braun

14. Schumacher G, Braun A, Kratzat R, Fabricius K, Roesler H, Plaue R (1982) Zur Anti-
    biotikumdiffusion aus dem Fibrin-Gentamycin-Verbund. In: Parsch K, Plaue R (Hrsg)
    Hämatogene Osteomyelitis und posttraumatische Osteitis, 28–31 Med Lit Verlagsgesellschaft,
    Uelzen 28–31
15. Ulatowski L, Goymann V, Meier M, Thümler P (1980) In-vitro-Ausdiffusion aus einem Fibrin-
    Antibiotika-Verbund. Orthop Praxis 10: 831
16. Ulatowski L, Meier M. Goymann V, Thümler P (1982) Pharmakokinetik eines Fibrinan-
    tibiotikumverbundes. In: Cotta H, Braun A (Hrsg) Fibrinkleber in Orthopädie und
    Traumatologie. Thieme, Stuttgart 196–199
17. Wahlig H, Dingeldein E, Braun A, Kratzat R (1982) Fibrinkleber und Antibiotika-Unter-
    suchungen zur Freisetzungstechnik. In: Cotta H, Braun A (Hrsg) Fibrinkleber in Orthopädie
    und Traumatologie. Thieme, Stuttgart 182–187
18. Zilch H, Drehsen R, Lambiris E, Hahn H (1982) Diffusionsverhalten von Cefotaxim aus der
    Fibrin-Antibiotika-Plombe im Tierversuch. In: Cotta H, Braun A (Hrsg) Fibrinkleber in
    Orthopädie und Traumatologie. Thieme, Stuttgart 191–195

Long-Term Results with the Use of Homologous Spongiosa Grafting in Connection with Fibrin Sealant in the Treatment of Chronic Osteomyelitis

W. Lack, P. Bösch, and H. Arbes

Key words: chronic osteomyelitis, homologous packing of foci, fibrin spongiosa grafting

Abstract

We report on the results of 29 cases of chronic osteomyelitis. Therapy consisted of extirpation of the focus and of filling of the cavity with homologous cancellous bone grafts using fibrin sealant. The anamneses of osteomyelitis ranged from 1 month to 42 years. We saw two cases of recidives both with giant osteomyelitic bone defects and high inflammatory activity. In one of those cases we were able to lower the inflammatory activity before surgery and achieve healing of the osteomyelitis. The excellent clinical results are attributed to the use of fibrin sealant in connection with specially prepared defattened and deantigenized homologous cancellous bone grafts. Employing the fibrin sealant improves the vascularization of the bone grafts and causes a slower release of the admixed antibiotic.

Results presented here show that excellent outcomes of treatment can be achieved in cases of chronic osteomyelitis using fibrin sealant only without additional autologous bone plasties.

Introduction

The choice of transplant for the packing of bone defects is still widely under discussion. Many authors contest the osteoinductive potency of nonautologous bone material and reject the use of homologous or heterologous cancellous bone grafts. Cases with poor osseous beds, as for example osteomyelitis, are considered especially uninviting [5, 6]. The additional incision, the increased postoperative morbidity, the weakening of the donor situs and the usually small amount of cancellous bone are the main disadvantages of using autologous bone material especially in cases of reoperation. The introduction of fibrin sealant seems to make up for the disadvantages of nonautologous implants as experimental research has shown that the ingrowth and remodeling of the graft is accelerated and improved [2, 3, 4]. The delayed release of the admixed antibiotic as well as the diminished growth of germs in the fibrin clot are the main reasons for choosing fibrin sealant as an antibiotic carrier in cases of chronic osteomyelitis.

Fibrin Sealant in Operative Medicine
Traumatology and Orthopaedics – Vol. 7
Edited by G. Schlag, H. Redl
© Springer-Verlag Berlin Heidelberg 1986

Material and Method

Twenty-nine cases of focus extirpation and packing in 28 patients with chronic osteomyelitis have been included in the study from 1975 to 1981. The 22 male and 6 female patients had an average age of 32 years (9 – 70 years). Osteomyelitis history ranged between 1 month and 42 years with an average of 12 years; 16 patients had undergone between one and five previous operations, mainly suction – through drainage or antibiotic instillations. The most frequent pathogen was *Staphylococcus aureus*. Four cases of Brodie's abscess, six of hematogenic osteomyelitis and 19 of posttraumatic osteomyelitis made up the collective. Seventeen of our patients had between one and four fistulas. For exact location of the foci see Table 1. Average follow – up was 55 months (36–94 months). All patients with a minimal follow-up of 3 years were included in the study.

Three main points are important in the clearing out of a focus. Firstly the fenestration of the corticalis has to be sufficiently large, the chiseling or reaming of the necrotic bone has to be done exactly and the medullary space has to be opened to gain access to the blood supply from the bone marrow. Packing of the defect is done with homologous bone grafts, which have been prepared in our own bone bank. Cancellous bone grafts are obtained from the metaphyses of distal femora and proximal tibiae from corpses. The chips to the size of approximately $0.5 \times 0.5 \times 3.0$ cm are then cleaned in a jet stream and defatted in a series of ether-alcohol solutions. The last rinsing is done with an antibiotic solution from which the chips are lyophilized in a high vacuum. After the final irradiation with cobalt-60 the chips can be stored at room temperature.

After having successfully cleaned the focus the surgeon proceeds to cut the bone chips to about pea size, sprinkles them with an antibiotic, mixes them with the fibrin sealant and inserts them in the cavity after having introduced the calcium-thrombin solution without the aprotinin. The cavity should be packed loosely to preserve the structure of the cancellous grafts. In between the layers of bone chips a soaking with the thrombin solution ensues. Because of the effect of the glue the implant can be

Table 1. Location of osteomyelitic foci

Tibia:	15 foci	Proximal epimetaphyseal part	1
		Proximal diametaphyseal part	5
		Proximal diaphyseal part	1
		Middiaphyseal part	3
		Distal diaphyseal part	5
Femur:	10 foci	Neck of femur	1
		Greater trochanter	2
		Proximal diaphyseal part	1
		Middiaphyseal part	1
		Distal diaphyseal part	2
		Distal diametaphyseal part	3
Calcaneum:	3 foci	Tuber calcanei	2
		Corpus calcanei	1
Humerus:	1 case	Proximal metaphyseal part	1

shaped at will and haemostasis is remarkable. After completion of the packing the periosteum and the muscles are glued with fibrin sealant and a superficial Redon drain is inserted if necessary.

Discussion

The packing of osteomyelitic defects with homologous cancellous bone grafts has shown excellent long-term results. The fibrin sealant system causes accelerated vascularization of the implant on the one hand and a delayed release of the antibiotic from the fibrin-bone graft mixture [7] on the other. It has also been proven to reduce the growth of pathogens in the implant as compared with the growth in the peripheral blood [8]. These properties of fibrin sealant even permit successfull packing of osteomyelitic foci with heterologous bone grafts [1]. This is especially remarkable as osteomyelitic foci have to be considered very unfavorable osseous beds for transplants because of the reduced vascularization, the frequently severe sclerosis and the fibrosis of the surrounding soft tissues.

The fact that both of the recurrences we saw occurred in the first couple of months following surgery and the good radiological incorporation of most of the implants at follow-up lead us to expect no further significant increase of recurrences. It is, however, not permissible to speak of complete healings in the cases with remaining sclerosis, as reexacerbations of the infections have been seen after many years when sequestrations or major sclerosis remain. Analysis of the two recurrences shows that both of them had a very high inflammation rate with blood sedimentation rates of 63/105 and 72/135 respectively (Westergreen method). Both foci were extremely large. Lowering the inflammatory activity with high-dose parenteral antibiotic treatment made it possible to achieve a permanent success after a second packing of the focus. This is the reason why we prefer a two-timed approach. After initial extirpation of the focus we now treat cases of osteomyelitis with high inflammation rates locally and systemically with antibiotics until the inflammatory parameters are significantly reduced. Only then do we proceed to pack the cavities with homologous bone grafts.

We believe that our positive experiences permit us to replace autologous spongiosa plasties with homologous fibrin-spongiosa plasties even in cases of chronic osteomyelitis with very disadvantageous starting points.

Results

The criteria for the assessment of healing were the clinical picture, the radiologically judged incorporation and remodeling, as well as the normalized blood sedimentation rate. With the exception of one sole case all foci packed have healed in blandly at follow-up. One patient complains about minor nocturnal pains, two have slight pains after extensive walking, and six suffer from minimal sensitivity to weather changes. The other 18 patients are completely free of complaints. Two recurrences after the 29 packings of foci were seen. Both cases had extremely large and fistulating defects of the distal femur in one patient and the proximal tibia in the other. Both of them had greatly increased blood sedimentation rates and the recurrence occurred within 6 months after the packing. The removal of the bone graft after a high-dose antibiotic treatment and subsequent renewed packing with homologous cancellous bone succeeded in bringing about healing of the infection in

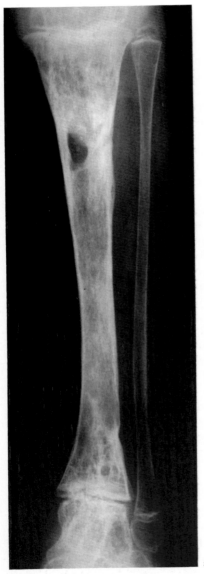 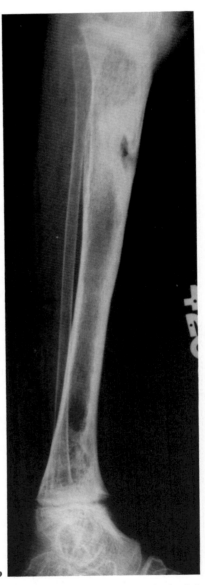

a   b

Fig. 1 a–d. Nine-year-old boy, posttraumatic polytope fistulating osteomyelitis, focus in the left proximal tibia, bacteriology, *Pseudomonas. c, d.* State 52 months following packing of the focus; free of pain, blood sedimentation rate normalized; radiological reconstruction of all structures, minor defect in the corticalis; result, "very good"

one case. The second patient – a 55-year-old man – is still suffering from his osteomyelitis.

The radiological evaluation shows a restitutio ad integrum in three cases with a complete restoration of the previous bone structure without any osseous scars. Thirteen cases with minor structural changes existed which were judged as very good (Figs. 1a-d). The incorporation and remodeling of more than two-thirds of the graft

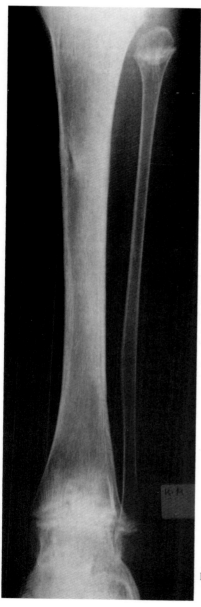

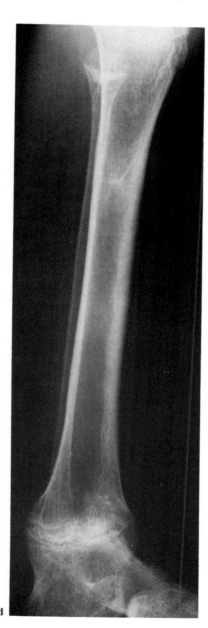

Fig. 1c

Fig. 1d

or the homogeneous sclerosation and complete incorporation with minor sclerotic islands was judged a good result in another 11 cases.

Because the incorporation of the cancellous bone grafts largely depends upon the operation technique, the age of the patient, the size of the focus as well as upon its location in relation to the meta- and diaphysis an exact description of the incorporation and remodeling processes is extremely difficult. A detailed analysis of our X-rays proved that small foci in cancellous regions like the calcaneum need about 6–12 months for complete incorporation of the transplanted bone bank grafts. The remodeling of medium-sized grafts in the tibia takes between 14 and 20 months, while our largest focus (about 40 cm^2) after 43 months is still not completely remodeled in its central areas. The recanalization of the medullary cavity can usually be seen after 20–24 months after medium-sized foci.

References

1. Arbes H, Bösch P, Lintner F, Salzer M (1981) First clinical experience with heterologous cancellous bone grafting combined with the fibrin adhesive system (FAS). Arch Orth Traumat Surg 98: 183-188
2. Bösch P, Braun F, Eschberger J, Spängler HP (1976) Experimentelle Untersuchungen über die Anwendung des "Fibrinklebesystems" bei der Knochenheilung. Forum f Exp Medizin Österr Ärztekongreß Wien 1976
3. Bösch P, Lintner F, Arbes H, Brand G (1980) Experimental investigations of the effect of the fibrin adhesive on the Kiel heterologous bone graft. Arch Orthop Traumat Surg 96: 177
4. Bösch P (1981) Die Fibrinspongiosaplastik; Experimentelle Untersuchungen und klinische Erfahrung. Wr Klin Wschr 93: 11 Supplement
5. Burri C (1974) Autologe Spongiosaplastik; In: Plane R: Die Behandlung der sekundär-chronischen Osteomyelitis; Bücherei des Orthopäden Band 13 1974, Enke Stuttgart.
6. Schweiberer L (1968) Experimentelle Untersuchungen von Knochentransplantation mit unveränderter und mit denaturierter Knochengrundsubstanz. Z Orthop 105: 465-484
7. Stanek G, Bösch P, Weber P, Hirschl A (1980) Experimentelle Untersuchungen über das pharmakokinetische Verhalten verschiedener, lokal applizierter Antibiotika im Knochen. Acta Med Austr Suppl 20: 19
8. Stanek G, Bösch P, Weber P (1980) Über die Keimmehrung in einem Fibrin-Klebesystem im Vergleich zu Blut und das Lyseverhalten mit und ohne Faktor XIII; in Fibrinogen, Fibrin und Fibrinkleber (Schimpf K. Husa) 239, Stuttgart New York; FK Schattauer 1980

The Mixture of Fibrin Sealant and a Porous Ceramic as Osteoconductor: An Experimental Study

J. PALACIOS-CARVAJAL and E. M. MOINA

Key words: Fibrin sealant, porous ceramic, osteoconduction

Abstract

Surgically created defects in rabbit femurs and iliac crests have been filled with a reabsorbable mixture of fibrin sealant and a porous tricalcium phosphate ceramic (TPC), in granular form. In another group only ceramic was implanted. Empty bone defects have been used as controls. Studies were performed, using histological techniques, 2 and 5 days, and 1, 2, 4, 8, and 12 weeks after implantation. The mixture is well tolerated by recipient tissues, with no untoward tissue reaction appearing. The process of implant replacement begins with the ingrowth of loose connective tissue rich in vessels. After 2 weeks osteoid tissue is found directly deposited on the TP particles' surface. During the following weeks the ceramic is gradually reabsorbed and replaced by lamellar bone. Bone ingrowth was usually observed within the ceramic pores greater than 100 µm wide. At 12 weeks after implantation, the cortex has almost completely been restored, the ceramic has been partially reabsorbed, and the marrow reestablished.

The results of this preliminary study indicate that the addition of fibrin sealant improves the osteogenetic capacity of an implant and that the mixture of fibrin sealant and TPC acts as a good osteoconductor.

Introduction

During the past few years, we have been using fibrin sealant in our Department of Traumatology and Orthopaedic Surgery. The mixture of fibrin sealant with autologous bone chips is used by us for filling bone defects or inserting different arthrodeses. Recently, calcium phosphate ceramic materials, which were developed for dental surgery, have been used for bone replacement in traumatology [4-7, 9]. These materials are dense or pourous forms of β-tricalcium phosphate and hydroxyapatite. They are available in powder, block, or granular forms of different sizes; frequently they have varied degrees of porosity ranging from macro (pores greater than 100 µm) to micro (pores less than 5 µm), created when the powder particles are not completely fused during the fabrication process.

It has been demonstrated that the biodegradable tricalcium phosphate implants are substituted by host bone tissue. The incorporation time is directly related to the implant size and the ceramic form chosen. The results of numerous experimental and clinical studies [1-3, 8, 10] reveal that all grafts are inproved by the addition of fibrin sealant. The exogenous fibrin produces adhesion, promotes tissue proliferation and vascularization, and improves the implant remodelling. The purpose of this experimental study has been to evaluate the effectiveness of a mixture of porous tricalcium phosphate ceramic (TPC) with fibrin sealant.

Materials and Method

Surgically created defects in the femurs and iliac crests of 22 rabbits were filled with a reabsorbable mixture of fibrin sealant and TPC. Similar defects were left empty as controls. In another group only bioceramic was implanted. The rabbits were killed sequentially 2 and 5 days, and 1, 2, 4, 8, and 12 weeks after implantation.

The mixture was prepared from 0.5 cc of fibrin sealant mixed with 1 g of tricalcium phosphate ceramic, i.e. 50% by volume of each component. The porous ceramic material we employed, in granular form, is produced from calcium phosphate powder by isostatic pressing. Then it is sintered at temperatures between 1100°C and 1300°C to produce a single-phase β-tricalcium phosphate. The powder is mixed with naphthalene, which evaporates during the sintering process, leaving a uniform distribution of large interconnecting pores inside the ceramic ranging from 100 to 300 μm in size. The final product has 36% porosity and a particle size ranging from 450 to 2000 μm. The fibrin sealant used consisted of a rabbit sealer protein concentrate and thrombin (4 IU/ml). We added the fibrinolysis inhibitor, Aprotinin (3000 KIU/ml).

The rabbits were killed at different times by an overdose of anesthetic, and the femurs and iliac crests removed. Blocks of tissue containing the implants were fixed in 10% buffered formalin. After fixation, they were decalcified; 4 μm sections were cut, stained with hematoxylin-eosin and Masson trichromic, and examined histologically.

Results

The histological behavior of TPC implants in combination with fibrin sealant showed a common sequence of events in the femur as well as in the iliac crest. Within the first few days after implantation, the implant was very quickly filled with a blood clot. The fibrin net included the TPC grains, penetrating more than 100 μm into the ceramic pores. Over the following days, the blood clot was reabsorbed; at the same time, loose connective tissue began to grow from the implant periphery. Although the methodology employed to fill the drill hole was the same in both groups of experiments (with and without fibrin sealant), the filling was better when we added fibrin sealant. Owing to its adhesive action, the mixture was easier to handle and the TPC particle distribution more uniform.

The complete implant was already infiltrated by connective tissue with fibroblasts and osteoblastic cells 1 week after implantation. The pattern of this connective tissue varied among the different groups of experiments, being denser when fibrin sealant was not added. The fibrin clot had been almost completely fibrinolyzed, even though we had added a fibrinolysis inhibitor. Revascularization had begun, and numerous vessels of small caliber could be observed through the fibrin-ceramic implant. Fibrous zones of increased density which are a preliminary stage of new metaplastic bone appeared, and osteogenic cells of the periosteum and of the endosteum had begun to proliferate. The presence of giant cells close to the ceramic grains at that stage represents a moderate foreign body response to the tricalcium phosphate, but this can be considered as minimal.

A well-developed callus rounded the injury zone 2 weeks after implantation (Fig. 1). Around the drill hole an area of devitalized bone, identifiable by the empty osteocyte lacunae, was produced by the heat generated during drilling and by the local destruction of the blood supply. In the group implanted with fibrin and ceramic, a dense network of osteoid tissue bridged the implant (Fig. 2), rounding each TPC particle; in the group implanted only with ceramic (Fig. 3), a narrow

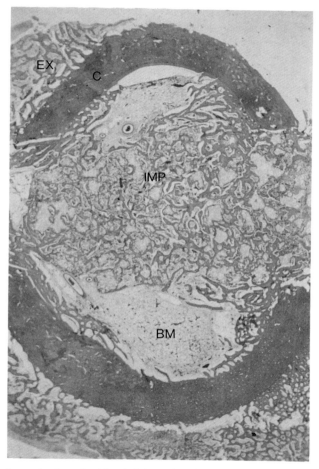

Fig. 1. Transverse section of a femur implanted with tricalcium phosphate ceramic and fibrin sealant, 2 weeks after surgery. *IMP,* Implant bridged by a net of osteoid tissue; *BM,* bone marrow; *C,* cortical bone; *EC,* external callus (HdE, x40)

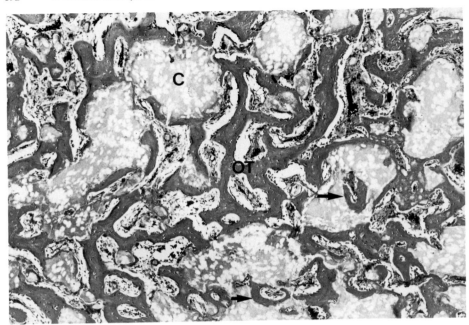

Fig. 2. A dense network of osteoid tissue (*OT*) bridges the implant of tricalcium phosphate ceramic in combination with fibrin sealant, 2 weeks after operation. *C.* tricalcium phosphate ceramic (HdE, × 100)

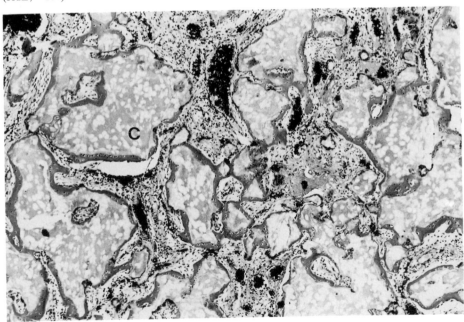

Fig. 3. After 2 weeks narrow deposits of osteoid tissue are rounding the ceramic grains (*C*) in the group implanted only with tricalcium phosphate ceramic (HdE, × 100)

osteoid deposit partially covered the ceramic grains. In a previously determined zone placed in the center of the implant, we measured the area occupied by the osteoid tissue. The results show that there was approximately twice the osteoid tissue in the group with the fibrin sealant implant , than in the group with only ceramic implant. Ingrowth of osteoid tissue was seen not only between and around the ceramic grains, but also inside the macropores (Fig. 4). This proliferating bone tissue was found deposited directly on the grain surface without the presence of any intervening tissue layer; numerous osteocytes living in close contact with tricalcium phosphate have been observed (Fig. 5).

The presence of numerous giant cells 4 weeks postimplantation (Fig. 6) is related to the ceramic reabsorption process. As the tricalcium phosphate dissolves in physiological solutions, the implant undergoes a passive chemical dissolution in addition to the cell-mediated process. As a result of deposits on the ceramic grain surface and inside the pores, osseous bridges are formed through the TPC particles (Fig. 7). Consequently, the particles are fragmented, and afterwards, the small pieces are phagocytosed by giant cells. In this way the ceramic is reabsorbed. At that stage, the first normally structured bone marrow could be identified through the implant placed in the medullary cavity in the nonfibrin-containing group, while in the fibrin-containing group bone marrow in the periphery had developed.

During the following weeks, the implant remodelling continued. The type of formed bone changed; earlier it was of the immature type, but later lamellar bone of the mature type was formed. Successive layers of new bone were deposited, converting cancellous bone into a more compact bone, which included some small ceramic pieces (Fig. 8). The osseous density differed between the implants with and

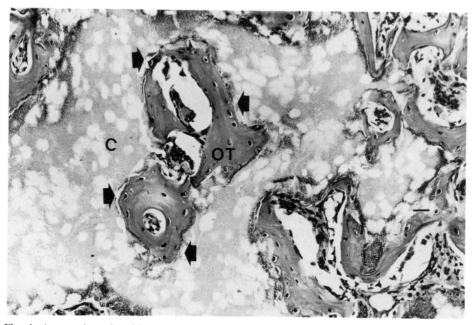

Fig. 4. A ceramic grain with a central macropore (*arrows*) greater than 100 μm, infiltrated by osteoid tissue (*OT*) (HdE, × 250)

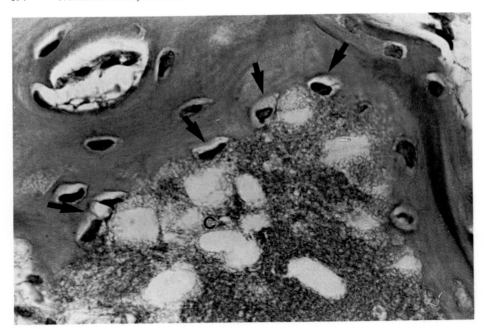

Fig. 5. Osteocytes *(arrows)* in close contact with the tricalcium phosphate ceramic *(C)*. (Masson trichromic stain, × 1000)

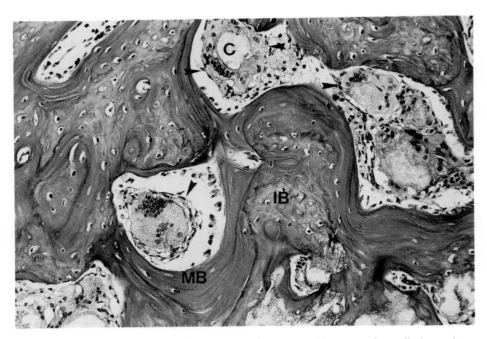

Fig. 6. Implant placed in cortical femur, 4 weeks after surgery. Numerous giant cells *(arrows)* are reabsorbing small ceramic pieces *(C)*. *IB* Immature bone; *MB*, mature bone (HdE, × 250)

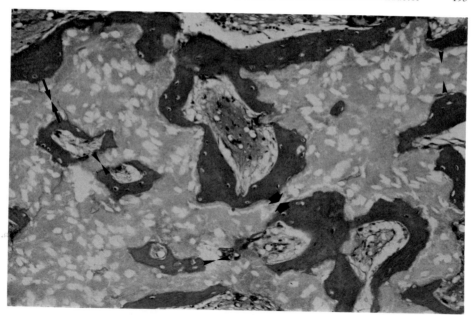

Fig. 7. Osseous bridges *(arrows)* formed through a ceramic grain. Implantation time was 8 weeks previously (Masson trichromic stain, × 250)

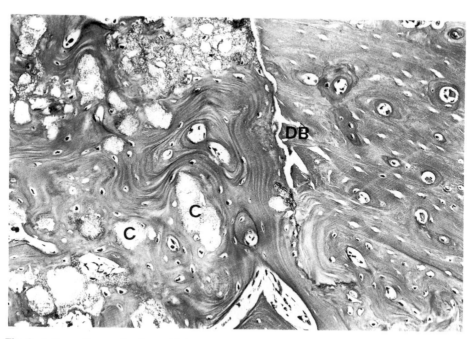

Fig. 8. *Left,* small ceramic pieces *(C)* included in compact bone; *right,* a zone of devitalized bone *DB)* remains 8 weeks after surgery (HdE, × 250)

without fibrin sealant, and this continued to be evident; in the appropriate locations the presence of more hematopoietic marrow could be observed.

After 12 weeks the cortex had been almost completely restored in the fibrin-ceramic group, while in the control group the cortical remodelling process was delayed, and bone continuity was not evident. Hematopoietic marrow occupied the medullary cavity, although bone trabeculae surrounding some TPC grains still remained in this area. The ceramic quantity was considerably reduced by reabsorption compared to the 8 weeks that at stage; the degradation rate of calcium phosphate as used was approximately 50% within the time duration of this experiment.

Variants of this process occurred depending on the type of bone repaired and the implant size. The healing of the iliac crest defects was faster than that of the femur defects, but the ceramic reabsorption was slower in the iliac crest. The surgical procedure was another factor that influenced host behavior and the way in which the implant was biodegraded. When the ceramic remained implanted in soft tissue with no exposure to freshly bleeding bone, the implant was quickly rounded by fibrous tissue. The ceramic reabsorption proceeded slowly. The pore size became enlarged through gradual dissolution and small pieces of ceramic were phagocytosed by multinucleated giant cells. This process continued slowly without any evidence of osteogenesis.

Discussion

There are many factors which must be considered when determining whether calcium phosphate ceramics are suitable as "bone graft substitutes". The principal limitation of these materials is their mechanical properties. They are quite brittle, have low impact resistance, and exhibit relatively low tensile strength [7]. However, they are composed of calcium and phosphate ions, the same ions of natural bone mineral, and are therefore well tolerated by the host tissue, not giving rise to any untoward tissue reaction.

On the other hand, the calcium phosphate implant materials are infiltrated and replaced by new bone, at the same time as they are reabsorbed. According to our results, a ceramic with interconnecting pore structure acts as a reabsorbable scaffold for the ingrowth of new bone. A minimal pore size is necessary to allow ingrowth of bone; we have not found bone infiltrating pores less than 100 μm wide.

The bone is directly deposited on the ceramic without any intervening tissue. The bonding zone probably evidences a chemical nature, but the details of its formation and the exact chemical composition of the "cementing" material are not yet fully understood [7].

The chemical composition, crystal structure, implant size, porosity, and other factors affect the degradation rate of the reabsorbable ceramic. There is considerable controversy on the question of the degradation rate. Some ceramic types are reabsorbed and some not at all or only partially; some are reabsorbed too fast and some too slow. A long-term experiment will be required to discover how long it takes for the TPC used here to be completely reabsorbed; nevertheless 50% of the initial implant had disappeared during the 12 weeks of this experiment.

It has been demonstrated [1-3, 8, 10] that fibrin sealant improves the incorporation of various types of graft. We have been able to verify that there is a similar advantageous action when synthetic tricalcium phosphate is used as a graft. The increase of bone ingrowth in the group implanted with both ceramic and fibrin sealant can be explained by an improvement of the osteogenic capacity, due to accelerated revascularization of the implant, by the addition of fibrin sealant.

Finally, we can conclude that the mixture of fibrin sealant with TPC acts as a good osteoconductor; it is very quickly infiltrated by new bone, gradually reabsorbed, and replaced by bone. The regenerated bone assumes the shape, conformity, and type of the original bone.

References

1. Arbes H, Bösch P, Lintner F, Salzer M (1981) First clinical experience with heterologous cancellous bone grafting combined with the fibrin adhesive system (FAS). Arch Orthop Trauma Surg 98: 183-188
2. Bösch P, Lintner F, Braun F (1979) Die autologe Spongiosatransplantation unter Anwendung des Fibrinklebersystems im Tierexperiment. Wien Klin Wochenschr 91: 628-633
3. Bösch P, Lintner F, Arbes H, Brand C (1980) Experimental investigations of the effect of the fibrin adhesive on the Kiel heterologous bone graft. Arch Orthop Trauma Surg 96: 177-185
4. Cameron HU, Macnab I, Pilliar RM (1977) Evaluation of a biodegradable ceramic. J Biomed Mater Res 11: 179-186
5. de Groot K (1980) Bioceramics consisting of calcium phosphate salts. Biomaterials 1: 47
6. Ferraro JW (1979) Experimental evaluation of ceramic calcium phosphate as a substitute for bone grafts. Plast Reconstr Surg 63: 634
7. Jarcho M (1981) Calcium phosphate ceramics as hard tissue prosthetics. Clin Orthop 157: 259–278
8. Lintner F, Bösch P, Arbes H, Brand G, Braun A (1982) Experimentelle Knochentransplantation. In: Cotta H Braun A (eds) Fibrinkleber in Orthopädie und Traumatologie: 4. Heilderberger Orthopädie-Symposium. Thieme, Stuttgart, pp 56–61
9. Uchida A, Nade S, McMartney E, Ching W (1984) The use of ceramics for bone replacement. A comparative study of three different porous ceramics. J Bone Joint Surg 66-B: 269-275
10. Zilch H (1982) Der Einfluß des Fibrinklebers auf die Revaskularissierung des Knochentransplantates. In: Cotta H Braun A (eds) Fibrinkleber in Orthopädie und Traumatologie: 4. Heidelberger Orthopädie-Symposium. Thieme Stuttart pp 62-64

The Combination of Fibrin Sealant (Tissucol/Tisseel) with Hydroxyapatite in Bone Surgery

E.C.MARINONI, M. ULIVI, and G.BONFIGLIO

Key words: Tissucol, hydroxyapatite, bone surgery

Abstract

In order to test the biocompatibility of a mixture of Tissucol with hydroxyapatite (in the form of crystallized powder mixed with Tissucol in equal parts) in relation to bone tissue, the following experiment was conducted in 16 New Zealand rabbits in the Orthopaedic Clinic of Milan. With the animals under general anaesthesia we drilled four holes, each 4 mm in diameter, in the femur and tibia. Each rabbit therefore had two femoral holes and two tibial holes, one in the diaphyseal and one in the metaphyseal segment, in both the right and left leg. We filled the holes with Tissucol, two with a combination of Tissucol-hydroxyapatite, and two with a mixture of Tissucol and *Kiel*-bone, while leaving the last two to heal spontaneously. After 7, 14, 20, 30 and 40 days the rabbits where killed under general anaesthesia; then radiographic and histological tests were performed.

In short we think that the association of Tissucol with hydroxyapatite can be a good method for repair of bone defects. In fact we are of the opinion that both elements of the mixture present good biocompatibility in relation to bone tissue. The radiographic and histological tests confirm this opinion.

Introduction

The aim of this research is to demonstrate the biocompatibility of a mixture of Tissucol and hydroxyapatite in relation to bone tissue when used to fill experimentally induced bone defects. We have also studied the evolution of bone holes when filled with the mixture of Tissucol-hydroxyapatite compared with those results obtained with the use of a mixture of Tissucol and *Kiel-bone* and with the use of Tissucol alone [1].

Material and Methods

Sixteen New Zealand rabbits were used in our experimental work. Four holes each 4 mm in diameter were made in the femur and in the tibia of all the animals under general anaesthesia.

Fibrin Sealant in Operative Medicine
Traumatology and Orthopaedics – Vol. 7
Edited by G. Schlag, H. Redl
© Springer-Verlag Berlin Heidelberg 1986

The holes were made either in the diaphysis or in the metaphysis in both right and left legs of each experimental subject. Subsequently two holes were made in the right femur as a control procedure while two holes were drilled in the right tibia later filled with the mixture of Tissucol and *Kiel*-bone. The two holes in the left femur were filled with Tissucol, while the two holes in the left tibia were filled with the Tissucol-hydroxyapatite mixture. The animals were killed on the (7th, 14th, 20th, 30th and 40th days). Histological and radiographical examinations were then performed on all the previously treated bones.

Results

Control Group

The holes in the diaphysis and in the metaphysis of the right femur were evaluated by radiography on the 7th, 14th, 20th, 30th and 40th days. In this way it was possible to study the various stages of the healing process in time. The physiological healing process and its development over time in the control group were also followed by histological examination. In this case we noted the appearance of new bone in the holes.

Experimental Group with the Tissucol-hydroxyapatite Mixture

The holes made in the right tibia of the animals were filled with the mixture of Tissucol-*Kiel*-bone. The animals were subsequently killed and evaluated with the same procedures as applied to the control group. The healing processes evaluated by radiography in these holes were similar to those observed in the control group, even if a reaction of the bone was present in relation to the *Kiel*-bone. The process of healing of the holes was also followed by histological examination either on the 14th day or on the 20th day.

Tissucol Group

The holes made in the diaphysis and metaphysis of the left femurs were filled by Tissucol alone. Both holes were evaluated by radiography and by histological examinations after the animals were killed on the same days as the other groups. The healing process of osteolysis was followed by radiographic examination and was similar to that observed in the control group. In particular, normal healing was observed on the 40th day. Furthermore, a clear division from the bone and Tissucol with residual trabeculae was seen by histological examination on the 17th day.

Experimental Group with the Tissucol-Hydroxyapatite Mixture

The holes in the femur and in the tibia were filled with the mixture of Tissucol and hydroxyapatite. Histological and radiographic examinations were performed on the

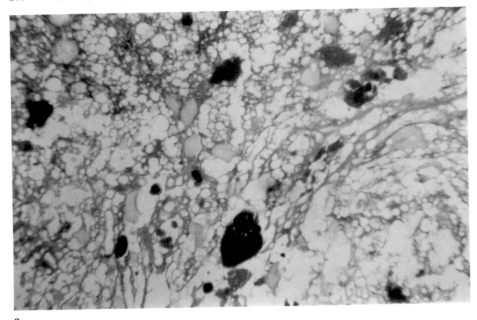

a

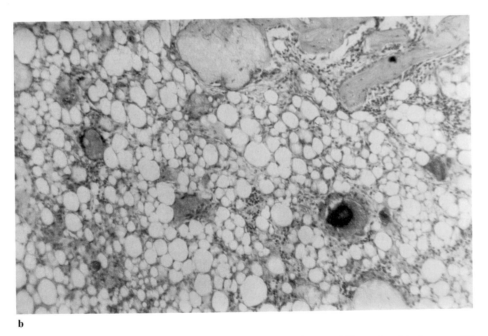

b

Fig. 1 a, b. A good integration of the bone tissue with the mixture of Tissucol and hydroxyapatite with the absence of inflammatory cells was seen on the 7th day *(a)*. Both elements of the mixture present good biocompatibility in relation to the bone tissue *(b)*.

same days as the other group. Radiographic examinations showed poor reactions of the bone towards the combination of Tissucol and hydroxyapatite. Healing of bone defects was deemed better than the healing seen in the group treated by Tissucol *Kiel*-bone. Good integration of the bone tissue with the mixture of Tissucol and hydroxyapatite with the absence of inflammatory cells was seen by histological examination on the 20th day, while the hydroxyapatite was integrated in the newly formed bone in particular on the 40th day (Fig. 1 a, b).

Conclusion

A complete recovery of bone in the experimentally induced holes was shown by the radiographic examinations performed on the 7th, 14th, 20th, 30th and 40th days. We would like to emphasize that radiographic examination showed that a combination of Tissucol with hydroxyapatite gave better results than the combination Tissucol-*Kiel*-bone or only Tissucol.

A complete recovery of bone in all the subjects examined was shown by the histological examination. Furthermore we believe that histological examination demonstrates that the mixture of Tissucol with hydroxyapatite is better than the associations Tissucol with *Kiel*-bone. The use of Tissucol is more useful in the healing of bone defects until the 10th-20th day; after this period its value in assisting the healing process is equal to that of the other groups. We think finally that the association of Tissucol and hydroxyapatite can be a good method to repair bone defects. In fact we believe that both elements of the mixture present a good biocompatibility in relation to the bone tissue.

References

1. Marinoni EC et al (1984) Proprietà biologica verso l'osso della associazione colla di fibrina ed idrossiapatite. Il Policlinico Sez Chirurgica 91: 1588-1591

The Influence of Fibrin Sealant and Osteoconduction in Femoral Defect Fillings with Hydroxyapatite and Beta-Tricalcium Phosphate Granules in Rats

J.-P. POCHON

Key words: Fibrin sealant, osteoconduction, hydroxyapatite, beta-tricalcium phosphate

Abstract

Femoral defects in 26 male rats (Iva:SIV, Kisslegg) were filled with hydroxyapatite and beta-tricalcium phosphate granules. Morphometric analysis showed a slightly increased osteoneogenesis with fibrin sealant but occurring later than without fibrin sealant. The amount of newly formed bone was between 3% and 23% higher than without fibrin sealant.

Introduction

The replacement of bone with autologous, homologous and heterologous bone presents many problems: resorption and infection, quantitative limitation and unsatisfactory mechanical qualities [4]. Synthetic ceramics like hydroxyapatite (HA) and beta-tricalcium phosphate (TCP) have many advantages [3]. Resorption is very slow, there is no quantitative limitation, sterilization is very easy, biocompatibility is proved [2] and osteoconduction begins 1 week after implantation.

The good results with the fibrin-spongiosa implant [1] encouraged us to ascertain whether HA and TCP with fibrin sealant (FS) improve osteoconduction.

Material and Method

Twenty-six male rats (Iva:SIV, Kisslegg) were operated on as follows: After opening the femurs by drilling, the holes were filled with HA and TCP granules (Ceros 82). Each animal was treated with and without FS injection to compare the bone formation in the same animal. FS (Tissucol) was applied with 3000 KIU/ml aprotinin. All implants were marked by intraperitoneally injected oxytetracycline (50 mg/kg) 48 hours before the rats were killed. The histological examination was carried out by morphometric methods.

Abbreviations:
HA: Hydroxyapatite
TCP: Beta-Tricalciumphosphate
FS: Fibrin sealant

Fibrin Sealant in Operative Medicine
Traumatology and Orthopaedics – Vol. 7
Edited by G. Schlag, H. Redl
© Springer-Verlag Berlin Heidelberg 1986

Results

1. *Masson-Goldnerstaining:* Osteoconduction on HA with FS was reduced by 54% – 81% in the 1st – 4th weeks after implantation in comparison with the animals without FS. Only at 8 weeks the animals showed an increased osteogenesis of 18%. The cases with TCP showed similar results (Table 1).
2. *Ultravioletmicroscopy:* In femurs filled up with HA the area of the osteogenetic activity was about 12% higher with FS. Two weeks after implantation the increase was between 32% and 167% with FS. On the contrary, 4 and 8 weeks after implantation the osteogenesis diminished to 39% – 75% in all cases with administration of FS (Table 2).

Table 1. Osteoconduction of HA and TCP granules without and with FS (percentage of area)

Weeks after implantation	Hydroxyapatite		Tricalcium phosphate	
	Without FS	With FS	Without FS	With FS
1	30.5	16.5	12.9	9.7
2	10.9	8.8	10.4	12.0
4	15.6	12.3	17.9	13.3
8	9.7	11.4	24.6	13.4

Table 2. Incorporation of tetracycline as expression of osteoneogenesis in HA and TCP granules without and with FS (percentage of area)

Weeks after implantation	Hydroxyapatite		Tricalcium phosphate	
	Without FS	With FS	Without FS	With FS
1	35.7	40.0	28.2	–
2	11.6	31.0	15.5	20.4
4	24.1	17.2	22.3	8.7
8	19.3	14.4	30.1	15.9

Discussion

Bösch et al. [1] demonstrated that FS only has an increasing effect on vascularization and shows no proper osteoinductive effects. In addition inhibitors of fibrinolysis such as aprotinin can inhibit vascularization. Our results underline the hypothesis that FS with aprotinin inhibits osteogenesis. On the contrary, the fixation of tetracycline as a sign of osteogenetic activity is not suppressed but even increased in the 1st and 2nd weeks of implantation. This means that FS leads to an increased activity of osteoblasts and that this phenomenon cannot be maintained because of lack of vascularization inhibited by aprotinin. The modern literature cannot give an other explanation.

The clinical application of ceramic implants with fibrin sealant has not yet been made. Further experimental work must be done in order to compare the osteogenetic effect with different concentrations of aprotinin. On the other hand, clinically implanted TCP in cases of juvenile bone cysts showed excellent results.

References

1. Bösch P, Arbes H, Lintner F, Ramach W (1982) Erfahrungen mit der Fibrinspongiosaplastik, Thieme, Stuttgart, pp 84-85 (Fibrinkleber in Orthopädie und Traumatologie)
2. Geret V, Rahn BA, Mathys R, Perren SM (1983) Quantitative Analyse der in vivo Gewebsverträglichkeit von Hydroxylapatit Ceros 80. Hefte zur Unfallheilk 165:75
3. Metzger DS, Driskell TD, Paulsrud JR (1982) Tricalcium phosphate ceramic – A resorbable bone implant: review and current status. J Am Dent Assoc 105:1035-1038
4. Pochon JP (1982) The repair of congenital and acquired skull defects. J Pediatr Surg 17/1:31-36

Fibrin Spongiosa Grafting in Hip Joint Replacement by a Cement-Free Judet Prosthesis

N. Wolf, T. Herzog, and H. Beck

Key words: Judet prosthesis, fibrin tissue adhesive sealant, spongiosa graft

Abstract

The problem of applying "bone cement" for fixation of total hip joint endoprotheses has been discussed in detail in the literature and has led to the development of numerous cement-free prosthesis models. In our opinion, the significance of the fibrin glue consists in more rapid and certain healing in of the spongiosa graft. In this way, a permanent fixation of the prosthesis component is possible in a large proportion both in primary implantations and in exchange operations (even after clearance of infections) using the Judet prosthesis.

Introduction

At the surgical Division of Erlangen University Medical School, the prosthesis developed by Judet has been used since 1980 and implanted in 668 cases up to the end of 1983, of which 455 were primary implantations and 213 exchange operations.

In the development of his prosthesis, Judet assumed that the fusion with the bone is promoted by a porous surface and that permanent stability is attained once fixation has occurred. This was initially confirmed in animal studies, and later also by investigations of explanted prostheses. Especially in application of the Judet prosthesis, a good implant bed is necessary for secure fixation of the prosthesis components, but this is usually not necessary to the extent required, above all, in exchange operations. In these cases, an adequate implant bed can be created using spongiosa. In the case of primary implantations, autologous spongiosa can be used for this purpose. However, in exchange operations this is not available in the amount required. The use of homologous spongiosa will then be necessary. This is available in adequate amounts from our bone bank. For stabilization and fixation of the spongiosa, we have employed fibrin tissue adhesive sealant to an increasing extent.

Materials and Methods

In a report on the clinical application of the fibrin tissue adhesive sealant system in connection with spongiosa transplants to fill bone defects, Bösch et al. [1] have

Fibrin Sealant in Operative Medicine
Traumatology and Orthopaedics – Vol. 7
Edited by G. Schlag, H. Redl
© Springer-Verlag Berlin Heidelberg 1986

described an accelerated homogeneous fusion of the transplanted spongiosa. As further advatages, the hemostyptic and adhesive strength of the power tissue adhesive sealant as well as the plastic deformability of the fibrin spongiosa graft were emphasized.

For the safety of the recipient of the spongiosa graft, the presence of hepatitis must be ruled out in the donors of homologous spongiosa by serology and measurement of the transaminase activity in the serum. The spongiosa is also not used if irregular antibodies are detected. The blood group (according to the ABO system) and the Rhesus factor of the donor and recipient should be the same. In addition, potential donors are tested for the presence of the HTLV-III antibody. General experience has shown that homologous spongiosa can be conserved for an almost unlimited time. However, if used too soon after removal, the result appears to deteriorate. For this reason, if possible only spongiosa more than 2 weeks old should be used.

According to Schricker and Scheele [2] a raised incidence of hepatitis B or hepatitis non-A-non-B is not present in application of fibrin tissue adhesive sealant. Afterwards, one case of hepatitis non-A-non-B which may have been due to the sealant was notified in more than 3000 patients with fibrin tissue adhesive sealant application. With a corresponding investigation of the potential donors of the homologous spongiosa and use of commercially available fibrin tissue adhesive sealant, the risk for the recipient is thus extremely low.

Besides the occasional application of fibrin spongiosa grafting in primary implantations of Judet prostheses, especially in the region of the acetabular bed, we carry out exchange operations for infection or loosening of cemented hip prostheses exclusively using homologous spongiosa with fibrin glue. After removal of the prosthesis components and the old bone cement components, large bone defects generally occur, especially in the region of the acetabulum. Since adequate amounts of autologous spongiosa are not available in exchange operations, the defects which have arisen must be filled by homologous fibrin spongiosa grafts. Apart from filling bone defects, fibrin spongiosa grafts are also required for reconstruction of the acetabular roof and more rarely also for securing the anchorage of the shaft components. The spongiosa chips are first comminuted if necessary and then mixed with the fibrin glue. This results in a plastically moldable mass. After introduction of the spongiosa into the bone defect, this is modelled into the desired form and the respective prosthesis components are then introduced. The fibrin spongiosa graft permeates the pores of the prosthesis and promotes the fixation of the Judet prosthesis in the new implant bed.

In a few cases, a two-session procedure is necessary when the defects are too large. In Fig. 1a, a long-lasting acetabular slackening with large bony defects in the bed of the cemented-in acetabulum is found in a 60-year-old woman. The explantation of the prosthesis with subsequent fibrin spongiosa grafting from seven femoral heads led to an acetabular bed capable of carrying weight (Fig. 1b). In the second session, the Judet prosthesis was implanted (Fig. 1c). Figure 1d shows the situation after half a year. The patient has put full weight on the operated hip for up to 2 months at this time.

A two-session procedure is also indicated in exchange operations for infected total hip joint endoprostheses. In the first operation, the old prosthesis is removed

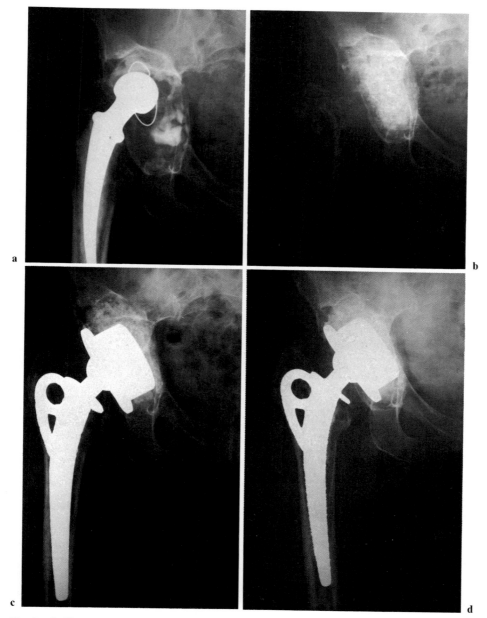

Fig. 1 a–d, X-ray sequence after an exchange of a total hip joint prosthesis in a 60-year-old female patient. *a* Initial situation. *b* Four months after prosthesis explantation and fibrin spongiosa grafting in the acetabular region, acetabular bed capable of carrying weight. *c* Immediate postoperative finding after implantation of a total Judet prosthesis once more with fibrin spongiosa grafting on the roof and base of the acetabulum. *d* Six months after operation, secure bony anchorage of the prosthesis acetabulum. (From [3])

Die Abbildung 1 a-d ist aus dem Buch "Fibrinklebung", herausgegeben von J. Scheele (Springer-Verlag) entnommen (S. 212)

together with the cement components and antibiotic-containing beads are inserted. After clearance of the infection, the implantation of the Judet prosthesis is carried out in the second operation. As a rule, a good-sized fibrin spongiosa graft is necessary here.

Results and Discussion

We were unable to observe a significant reduction of the postoperative loss of blood in application of fibrin spongiosa grafts as compared to operations not using fibrin. However, in contrast to other authors we do not seal the shaft and acetabular region with fibrin at the end of the operation.

We were able to check the rates of take of fibrin spongiosa grafts for a relatively standardized operation, namely the implantation of cement-free Judet prosthesis in exchange operations with in some cases appreciable bed defects in 113 cases from 1980 until 1983. After aseptic slackening, the Judet prostheses had become firmly fixed in 90% of the cases in which the operation had been more than 2 years prior to the time of follow-up examination. In cases of septic slackening, the prostheses were clinically and radiologically firm in 70%.

References

1. Bösch P, Lintner F, Braun F (1979) Die autologe Spongiosatransplantation unter Anwendung des Fibrinklebesystems im Tierexperiment. Wien Klin Wochenschr 91:628-633
2. Schricker KT, Scheele J (1984) Hepatitisrisiko der Fibrinklebung in der Allgemeinchirurgie. In: Scheele J (Hrsg) Fibrinklebung. Springer, Berlin Heidelberg New York Tokyo, pp 227-231
3. Wolf N, Scheele J, Link W, Beck H (1984) Die Fibrinspongiosaplastik beim Hüftgelenkersatz mittels zementfreier Judet-Prothesen. In: Scheele J (Hrsg) Fibrinklebung. Springer, Berlin Heidelberg New York Tokyo, p 212

Application of Fibrin Sealant and Transplantation of Allogeneic Bone in Traumatology and Joint Replacement

G. BLÜMEL, R. ASCHERL, F. LECHNER, and K. GEISSDÖRFER

Key words: Fibrin sealant, alloarthroplasty, bone allografts

Abstract

In addition to being used with frozen spongious bone allografts, fibrin sealant has been applied in the treatment of bone defects. Local hemostasis as well as the plasticity and better handling of the transplants are advantageous conditions when fibrin sealant is used. According to the final results the nontreated allografts are equal to those treated with fibrin; however in the early postoperative course radiological evaluation indicates a more rapid ingrowth of bone in the grafts treated additionally with fibrin.

The origin of transplantation surgery is closely connected with the transplantation of bone. Furthermore bone was the first tissue to be transplanted successfully following long-term preservation.

These preservation procedures, which have been applied already by Axhausen [1] and Lexer [5], have nowadays regained particular significance as

a) the number of comminuted open fractures and their sequelae is still increasing, and

b) in revision surgery of alloarthroplasties difficult problems are posed when loosening is accompanied by extended loss of bone.

Because of the additional extension of surgery, and the frequently advanced age of the patients, transplantation of autologous bone cannot always be easily performed. Following multiple surgery it is difficult to harvest a satisfying amount of autologous graft material.

Cryopreserved Allogeneic Bone

If there is insufficient quantity or quality of autologous bone grafts, a bone bank can provide an equivalent substitute. Centers specialized in joint replacement can easily maintain their own bone banks without any large financial or technical efforts. Our experiences and results derive from a close cooperation with the Garmisch-Partenkirchen Hospital, where spongious bone has been cryopreserved routinely for more than 4 years.

Donor bone is harvested from the femoral necks in cases of total hip joint replacement. Bone cysts, necrotic and sclerotic bone, as well as cartilage are

Fibrin Sealant in Operative Medicine
Traumatology and Orthopaedics – Vol. 7
Edited by G. Schlag, H. Redl
© Springer-Verlag Berlin Heidelberg 1986

removed. Then blocks 1 or 2 cm^3 in size are stored in air-proof glasses at a temperature of -90°C in an electric freezer under sterile conditions. Inflammatory diseases, such as hepatitis, lues, AIDS, and rheumatism, must be excluded in potential donors, so before freezing and after thawing (dry, at room temperature) swabs must be taken from the transplants.

The significance of cryopreserved spongious bone lies in the second phase of osteogenesis according to Axhausen [2]: the host tissue is stimulated by the nonvital transplant, i. e., metaplasia of the surrounding (soft) tissue occurs, which leads to bone formation at the surface of the allograft. True osteogenesis cannot be expected but is induced. Distinct alterations in the structure of the transplant's matrix following freezing below -90°C seem to be of particular importance for its osteoinductive capacity.

Fibrin Sealant and Bone Allografts

When using fibrin sealant as an auxiliary, one has to be aware of the comparatively high fibrinolytic activity of cryopreserved bone (Fig. 1). This can be demonstrated histochemically by fibrinolysis autographs according to Todd [9]. Cryo-cut histological specimens were incubated on a slide with a fibrin layer containing plasminogen and the size and depth of lysis estimated according to Pandolfi et al. [7].

Our findings suggest that a high concentration of aprotinin in the fibrin sealant acts as an antiprotease, protecting the fibrin from rapid lysis.

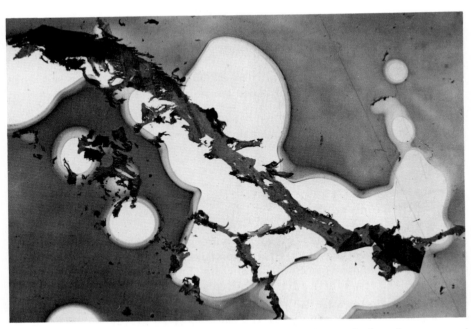

Fig. 1. Fibrinolysis autographs according to Todd with massive lysis around a thawed cryopreserved bone allograft. ×4.7

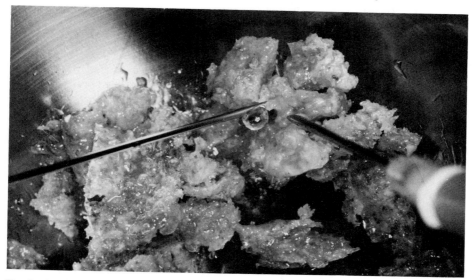

Fig. 2. Application of fibrin sealant on to thawed allogeneic bone chips

In principle the deep frozen fibrinogen is used with the thrombin compound of highly concentrated aprotinin.

The spongious bone is minced and, after complete thawing at room temperature, the sealant compounds are added to produce a homogenous mass of excellent plasticity (Fig. 2). Thus a good modelling of the transplant with special regard to the shape of the implantation site can be achieved. This gives the additional advantages of better blood clotting and initial fixation.

Chemical Materials and Methods

In 5 years 396 allogeneic transplantations have been performed. The majority of these cases (80%) were patients with excessive bone resorption with loosening of endoprostheses, the remaining 20% were patients with fresh fractures and nonunions.

Forty-nine patients, receiving 51 allogeneic transplants, underwent a prospective clinical trial: 27 bone grafts were transplanted without fibrin adhesive, while 24 transplants had fibrin sealant applied. The recipients were 67 years old on average; the mean age of donors was 62 years.

Radiographisies were evaluated according to a four point scale proposed by Kalbe [4]. In addition our own evaluation criteria were used: general bone formation, structure and resorption of the transplant were evaluated for a period of 6 months.

Clinical Results

According to the final results there were no differences between the two groups. Differences however could be demonstrated in the course of healing. There was a more rapid ingrowth and healing when fibrin sealant was included. The two following case reports demonstrate the value of using cryopreserved bone as well as that of fibrin sealant.

Case Reports

D.R.A.: an 85 year old female

This case demonstrates clearly the sometimes severe sequelae of joint replacements. Altogether four operations have been performed on this patient's right hip. Finally a septic loosening occurred in the femoral compartment of her right THR, with massive lysis of the lateral cortex of the proximal femur. Following local antibiotic treatment with pMMA-beats, a femoral prosthesis with a long stem was implanted and the defect area was filled with allogeneic spongious bone. To encourage better attachment the graft was treated with fibrin adhesive. Within 12 weeks a thin but continuous cortex was reestablished (Fig. 3).

W.M.: an 84 year old female

The spontaneous fracture in the proximal femur due to osteoporosis was treated primarily by plate fixation. This plate and the following implant failed because of fatigue fractures. The third operation involved internal fixation with the additional use of bone cement, filling the defect in the medial third of the upper femur with allogeneic bone and applying fibrin adhesive. In spite of the bad conditions and the age of the patient bony consolidation did occur (Fig. 4).

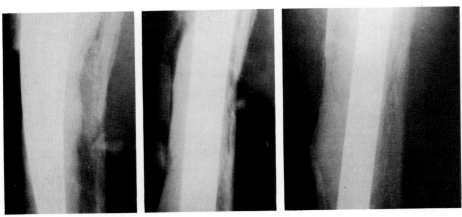

Fig. 3. Bony consolidation of an osseous defect following septic loosening of THR. The allogeneic bone has been attached by fibrin sealant (see case report)

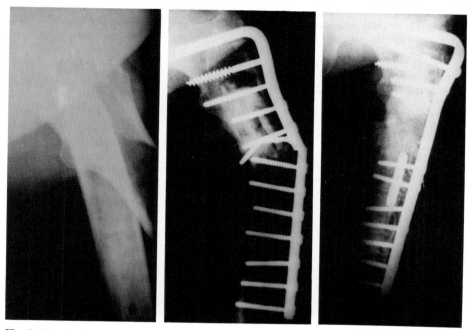

Fig. 4. Note healing of fracture in the upper femur following multiple surgery (see case report)

Conclusion

As in autologous bone grafts the advantages of simultaneous application of fibrin sealant include the initial immobilization of the bone graft and close contact with the host tissue [8]. Furthermore the blood clotting effect is very significant. Some reports indicate improved bone formation in the vicinity of even xenogeneic bone [3,6]. Thus the use of fibrin sealant makes handling and transplantation of allogeneic bone easier and seems to enhance the transplant's osteoinductive capacity.

References

1. Axhausen G (1909) Über den Vorgang partieller Sequestrierung transplantierten Knochengewebes nebst neuen histologischen Untersuchungen über Knochentransplantation an Menschen. Langenbecks Arch Chir 89: 281
2. Axhausen W (1952) Die Knochenregeneration – ein zweiphasiges Geschehen. Zentralbl Chir 77: 435
3. Bösch P. Lintner F, Arbes H, Brand G (1980) Experimental investigations of the effect of the fibrin adhesive on the kiel heterologous bone graft. Arch Orthop. Trauma Surg 96: 177-185
4. Kalbe P (1980) Die Transplantation allogener, kältekonservierter Hüftkopfspongiosa. Grundlagen, Indikationen, Technik und Ergebnisse, Thesis, Hannover

5. Lexer E (1924) Die freien Transplantationen, Enke, Stuttgart
6. Lintner F, Bösch P, Arbes H, Brand G, Braun F (1982) Experimentelle Knochentransplantation. In: Cotta H, Braun A (eds) Fibrinkleber in Orthopädie und Traumatologie. Thieme, Stuttgart, pp 56-61
7. Pandolfi M, Ahlberg A, Traldi N, Nilsson IM (1972) Fibrinolytic activity of human synovial membranes in health and in haemophilia. Scand J Haematol 9: 572-576
8. Stübinger B, Fritsche HM, Prokscha GW, Blümel G (1982) Die "Spongiosa-Fibrinkleber-Plombe" zur Überbrückung von Knochendefekten. Z Orthop 120: 445
9. Todd AS (1964) The histological localisation of fibrinolysin activator. J Pathol Bact 78: 281-283

Bone Banking and Fibrin-Adhesive System

G. Kellner, P. Bösch, and W. Ramach

Key words: Bone banking, homologous bone grafts, fibrin – adhesion system, fibrin – spongiosa grafting

Abstract

The one essential precondition for optimal remodelling of the graft after bone transplants is the ingrowth of blood vessels from the osseous bed. This means that the preparation technique is of overall importance when homologous bone chips are used. We present a method for production of bone grafts clean of cells and fatty tissue. The bone chips, which have been treated with water, ether and alcohol and have been lyophilized and irradiated, are, in combination with the fibrin-adhesion system, the optimal basis for vascular ingrowth and lack almost completely any antigenic potency. This technique improves the incorporation of the bone grafts significantly and also strongly reduces the rate of infection from 5% to 0.4% in sterile and from 36% to 6% in osteomyelitic cases.

Introduction

The fate of cancellous bone grafts in packings of bone defects is largely determined by access to the vascular system of the osseous bed. The vascularization depends upon the localization and the size of the defect, the patients age, the adaptation of the bone chips to their osseous bed and mechanical immobilization [8, 12]. Which kind of bone graft is used is highly relevant. Many assume that fresh autologous transplants are easily incorporated and remodelled because of their high osteogenic potency [1, 9, 13]. Most authors deny homologous and heterologous transplants any osteogenic potency, but concede that they can lead to osseous ingrowth of the packed defect via osteoinduction [2, 3, 7, 10]. The fibrin sealant is especially interesting in cases of bone transplants as blood vessels are known to grow along the fibrin grid of natural haematoma [5, 6, 11].

The following advantages of fibrin-spongiosa plasties have been proven [4]:
1. Optimum staunching of the bleeding and thus prevention of seroma
2. Plastic formability to render optimal shaping of the chips possible
3. Accelerated bony incorporation by means of improved vascularization via the fibrin grid
4. Improved retention of the admixed antibiotic

Fibrin Sealant in Operative Medicine
Traumatology and Orthopaedics – Vol. 7
Edited by G. Schlag, H. Redl
© Springer-Verlag Berlin Heidelberg 1986

The quality of the homologous cancellous bone is of essential importance for the osseous incorporation of the graft. The differences in attitude of the various authors towards homologous grafts stem mainly from differences in preparation techniques. "Homologous" usually means the use of freshly removed, deep frozen or even lyophilized bone, but rarely includes a defattening process. The non-defattened bones have various disadvantages. For one the fat is a mechanical obstacle for ingrowth of blood vessels and secondly the danger of an antibody-antigen reaction of the host versus the bone marrow of the donor is greatly increased.

Material and Methods

The Orthopaedic Clinic of the University of Vienna has been using its own bone bank since 1965 to prepare homologous cancellous bone chips [4, 8]. The chips are taken from the diaphyseal and metaphyseal parts of the proximal tibiae and distal femora of fatal accidents. The removal of the grafts has to take place not more than 6 h after the death and must be done under sterile conditions. Donors should be between 25 and 50 years of age. The large amount of endostal parietal cells strongly influences further processing in younger donors, while the high incidence of neoplastic and metabolic diseases of older people has to be taken into account. The material can be stored in a home-type mechanical freezer at $-15°$ to $20°C$ until processing. Usually bone chips of the size of $0.5 \times 0.5 \times 5$ cm are prepared.

Preparation Technique I (1965–1980)

The further processing of the chips was done until 1980 by lyophilizing them in vacuum at $-60°C$ with one short interruption to heat them to $+40°C$ to let the fat drip off the chips. The dried chips were then irradiated with cobalt-60 at 2.5 Mrad and stored in sealed glass jars.

Preparation Technique II (Since 1980)

Because defattening of the bone chips can only be achieved incompletely with a one-time heating, we have been carrying out the further processing as follows. The chips are firstly rinsed in flowing hot tapwater for 3–4 h to clean them mechanically. They are then introduced into a bath of ether for three times 3 h with two complete changes of the ether. To elute the ether we rinse the chips with a series of alcohol solutions of descending concentration. We begin with 70% alcohol, continue with 50% alcohol and finish with 20% alcohol within approximately 2 h. After a final bath in pure water we soak the chips in an antibiotic solution (neomycin and bacitracin) and introduce them into the glass jars in various amounts as needed for surgery. The lyophilization can be done either automatically or semiautomatically. The containers are then filled with pure nitrogen to obtain an absolutely dry environment and sealed with paraffin. The radioactive irradiation with 2.5 Mrad of cobalt-60 achieves the required sterility and denatures any remaining cellular contents among the bone chips and thus almost completely eliminates their antigenic potency [5, 8, 12].

Fibrin-Spongiosa Plug (Operation Technique)

The fibrin-spongiosa plug has been in use at the Orthopaedic Clinic of the University of Vienna since 1975 [4]. The preparation of the osseous defect is done as usual. The cleaning of the cavity has to be as radical as possible and sclerotic, badly vascularized bone tissue has to be chiselled away to reach healthy cancellous areas. The larger the opening into the bone marrow, the easier will be the ingrowth of new blood vessels into the graft. The bone chips are then prepared to about peasize and soaked with the fibrin sealant. We now introduce layer after layer of the fibrinogen-spongiosa mixture and spray them intermittingly with a concentrated calcium-thrombin solution. If possible we try to preserve the spongious structure of the chips. The approximate amount of fibrin sealant needed is usually arrived at using a simple formula: length × width of the defect divided by a specific quotient for every transplant. The quotient is 2.5 for lyophilized homologous chips, 3–3.5 for autologous grafts and 2 for the heterologous grafts.

This method guarantees an exact adaptation of the chips to their osseous bed and towards each other. The formation of cavities can so be avoided. Optimal haemostasis is one of the additional interesting features.

When used for packing of osteomyelitic defects the chips are routinely mixed with an antibiotic powder before addition of the fibrin sealant.

Because of the width of the defects we refrain from using aprotinin as it would obstruct fibrinolysis necessary for vascular ingrowth.

Indications and Results

In the period from 1965 to 1980 the Orthopaedic Clinic of the University of Vienna has used homologous cancellous bone grafts in 381 operations. From 1981 to March 1985 they have been employed in another 416. Indications can be seen in Table 1.

Table 1. Indications for implantation of Homologous cancellous bone until 1974 without FAS, from 1975 with FAS (except dorsal spondylodesis)

	1965–1980	1981 – March 1985
Tumours	119	102
Dorsal spondylodesis	226	96
Total hip-revision	–	136
Osteomyelitis	36	19
Others	–	63
Total	381	416

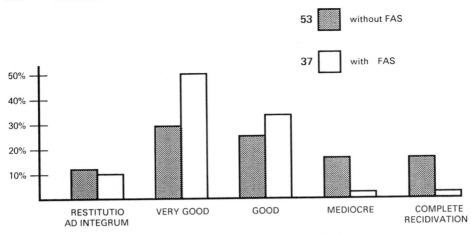

Fig. 1. X-ray results of homologous spongiosa plasties with lyophilized, irradiated non-defattened chips

With the sole exception of dorsal spondylodeses the fibrin adhesion system has been employed regularly since 1975.

The remodelling of transplanted cancellous bone has been significantly accelerated with the use of fibrin sealant because of faster vascularization. This has been shown in a comparative study between 37 cases with and 53 cases without the fibrin adhesion system (FAS). Figure 1 shows the radiological criteria of incorporation of the two groups.

Excellent results have been obtained in connection with infection rates. Reinfections were seen in only 6% of the cases in which the FAS was used as compared with 36% without after the packing of osteomyelitic foci. Non-septic defects had a rate of 4.6% without and 5.7% with FAS when non-defattened cancellous bone was used. We succeeded in lowering this rate to 0.4% with our improved preparation technique (see Table 2).

Table 2. Infection rate after implantation of homologous cancellous bone

Non-defattened		Defattened	
Without FAS ($n = 291$) 5.6%	With FAS ($n = 85$) 4.5%	Without FAS ($n = 165$) 0%	With FAS ($n = 338$) 0.4%

Discussion

Using the fibrin adhesion system in combination with well-prepared cancellous bone grafts has been very successful so far. The remodelling has been significantly improved with the fibrin sealant. The sclerosation of the central parts of the implant in cases of packing of major defects or osteomyelitic foci has been seen less frequently and to a much smaller degree.

The low rate of infections can be attributed in addition to the radical operation technique employed to the following factors:

1. The thorough packing of the defect with the fibrin-spongiosa mixture prevents the formation of seroma
2. The retention of the admixed antibiotic in the clot causes a slow and localized release
3. The cellular elements within the bone grafts are denatured and their antigenicity is completely eliminated after the exact cleaning

We cannot yet offer final long-term results about the incorporation of the defattened, lyophilized and irradiated cancellous bone grafts. Our observations especially of the significantly reduced rate of infections so far permit us to consider the refined preparation technique justified.

References

1. Andrew C, Basset L, Gibson Packard A Jr (1959) A clinical assay of cathode ray sterilized cadaver bone grafts. Acta orthop Scand 28, 198
2. Axhausen W (1954) Der biologische Wert heteroplastischer Knochentransplantate. Langenbecks Arch u Dtsch Z Chir 279, 48
3. Baadsgard K (1970) Kiel bone in the treatment of pseudarthrosis. Acta orthop Scand 40, 696
4. Bösch P (1984) Die Fibrinspongiosaplastik. Experimentelle Untersuchungen und klinische Erfahrungen. Wien klin Wschr 93, 11 Supll 124
5. Burwell RG (1966) Studies in the transplantation of bone. VIII. Treated composite homograft-autografts of cancellous bone: an analysis of inductive mechanisms in bone transplantation. J Bone Jt Surg 48B, 532
6. Dambe LT, Saur K, Schweiberer L (1978) Revascularisation frischer homologer Knochentransplantate in der Diaphyse des Röhrenknochens beim Hund. Arch Orth Traum Surg 92, 35
7. Hutchinson J (1952 The fate of experimental bone autografts and homograft. Brit J Surg 39, 552
8. Meznik F, Slancar P (1969) Klinische Ergebnisse auto-, homo- und heterologer Knochentransplantationen. Z Orthop 105, 465
9. Rathke FW (1965) Spongiosa-Implantation bei osteomyelitischen Trepanationshöhlen. Z Orthop 100, 218
10. Schweiberer L (1970) Experimentelle Untersuchungen von Knochentransplantaten mit unveränderter und mit denaturierter Knochengrundsubstanz. Unfallheilkunde, Suppl 103
11. Thielemann F, Veihelmann D, Schmidt K (1978) Die Induktion der Knochenneubildung nach Transplantation. Arch Orthop Traum Surg 91, 3
12. Vittali HP (1965) Die biologischen Grundlagen der Knochentransplantation. Z Orthop 99, 146
13. Witt AN (1965) Die operative Behandlung der Osteomyelitis. Z Orthop 100, Beilagenheft, 200

The Use of Fibrin Sealant (Tissucol) in Hemophilic Orthopedic Surgery

G. Torri, E. Lozej, P. Cerea, G. Mistò, R. Attolini, P. Molinari, F. Mapelli, W. Albisetti, and C. Micale

Key words: Hemophilia, fibrin seal, orthopedic surgery

Abstract

Our experience in the use of fibrin sealant in hemophilic patients undergoing operations for bone diseases has been acquired over many years. The main application has been filling hemophilic bone cysts and pseudotumors. In these cases, the clotting properties of Tissucol mixed with spongious bone implants have been shown to reduce postoperative bleeding and consequent relapse of the cyst. From these experiences we have received our first impressions of the effectiveness of "Tissucol" in tissue repair. Tissucol has also been used to cover exposed bone areas in hemophilics with factor VIII inhibitor. Furthermore, if substitutive therapy with factor VIII in the postoperative period of hemophilic patients has not been reduced in practice, the use of Tissucol has been shown to improve the quality of skin suture, so that the healing period (that in hemophilic patients is often lengthened) becomes quite normal.

Introduction

In early 1977, in our institute, we used for the first time frozen human fibrinogen mixed together with a little material from spongious bone grafts, to pack hemophiliac bone cyst of the proximal tibia; the aim was to make a close connection of the bone with the grafts [7]. The success of surgery in hemophilic patients depends primarily upon the adequacy of replacement therapy [2, 3]. Nevertheless the major problem in hemophiliacs undergoing orthopedic surgery, for example, for a bone cyst is the small vessel bleeding of the bone, because of the impossibility of achieving effective hemostasis in situ. In addition, in hemophilic cysts and pseudotumors there is a "membrane" which has to be taken off completely during the operation; otherwise it behaves as a filter, allowing a continuous flow of serum and blood toward the cavity. For this reason, we can say that the "cystic membrane" is very similar to the hyperplastic synovia in the histiocitic phase, often seen in hemophilic patients. The histological features explain why the surgery of a hemophiliac cyst (in the bone or in the muscle) and the surgery of the pseudotumors is often complicated by incomplete healing up of the wound, with presence of fistulas [8, 9]. The incidence of these complications has been significantly reduced by the use of human lyophilized fibrinogen, activated by thrombin, and injected into the cavity; the

Fibrin Sealant in Operative Medicine
Traumatology and Orthopaedics – Vol. 7
Edited by G. Schlag, H. Redl
© Springer-Verlag Berlin Heidelberg 1986

enzymatic conversion of fibrinogen in fibrin will occur in situ [1]. In this way a local hemostasis of the small vessel of the bone will be achieved and the small vessel bleeding controlled. Therefore, the Tissucol bypassing the major problem of the healing of the tissues, due to a slow formation of the clot, so that fibrin polymerization is impaired, aids effective local hemostasis. The problem of the healing of the wound due to a delay in clot formation is also present in other clotting defects, including thrombocytopathies. It is not very well known whether the specific clotting defect, i. e., factor VIII or factor IX deficiency, is the only reason for a delay in wound healing; so we cannot exclude that the fibronectin present in Tissucol may contribute to local cicatrization. In practice, Tissucol gives rise to an artificial but effective clot for about 5–7 days, so that physiological beginning of healing is favoured.

Materials, Methods and Case Histories

In the past 8 years we have used frozen or lyophilized Tissucol in 70% of orthopedic surgery in hemophiliacs. In nine operations of hemophilic cysts of the bone, located mainly at the tibial and femoral condyles, but also at the distal tibia, Tissucol has been used together with small grafts of spongious bone. In four hemophilic pseudotumors located at the thigh, calf, and femur, respectively, Tissucol has been used to fill the cavity resulting from the removal of the pseudotumors. Tissucol was also very effective in the control of small-vessel bleeding in patients with von Willebrand's disease, in whom the deficiency of factor VIII is associated with a prolonged bleeding time. In these patients fibrinogen has also been injected into bone drill holes resulting from screw removal after surgical treatment for fractures, because of the impossibility of achieving effective local hemostasis. Tissucol has also been added in tenorrhaphies, performed in four operations of Achilles tendon lengthening, and to strengthen the suture of the tendon sheath and of the skin. In three synovectomies of the knee, Tissucol has been placed at the insertion of the synovia to the bone of the femoral condyles. In two hemophilic patients with antibodies to factor VIII, Tissucol has been added to skin grafts to cover the exposed bone [4, 5]. Finally, in three hemophilic patients affected by a severe chondropathy of the patella and of the femoral condyles, Tissucol has been added in a thin layer on the patella surface after cartilage "shaving", and injected into the bone drill holes. Tissucol has also been used for direct injection to close postoperative skin fistulas.

In all the operations performed with Tissucol in hemophilic patients we always use a thrombin solution of 500 NIH/ml and an aprotinin solution of 3000 KIU/ml; Tissucol has often been mixed with spongious bone grafts, before inserting them into bone cyst, and it has often been applied before and after pneumatic tourniquet removal.

Results

From these experiences we can conclude that the advantages of using Tissucol in hemophilic surgery are:

1. The presence of fibronectin may in some way correct the biological defect arising from impaired clot polymerization.
2. Clotting properties reduce bone bleeding and the subsequent relapse in cysts and pseudotumors.
3. Tissucol has been shown to improve the quality of skin suture so that the healing period becomes quite normal.

Discussion

For all these reasons, we think that the future application of Tissucol in hemophilic patients will be: the percutaneous treatment of pseudotumors, the possibility of minor surgery in patients with factor VIII antibodies [4, 5] and the reduction in replacement therapy with factor VIII or IX after surgery [1].

In conclusion, we think that human lyophilized fibrinogen is a very important tool in ensuring the success of surgery in hemophiliacs; in fact with the use of Tissucol, we have also performed nonelective orthopedic surgery in hemophiliacs with antibodies to factor VIII.

References

1. Baudo F (1984) Applicazioni cliniche del Tissucol. clot hematol malignancies 1: 23–27
2. Bösch P, Lintner F, Nowotny Ch, Schwägerl W, Thaler E (1978) Operation eines hämophilen Pseudotumors unter Verwendung der Fibrinspongiosaplastik. Hämophilie-Symp, Hamburg 1977, Gilandbeck, Marx R (Hrsg), Global Druck u. Verlag, Heidelberg 289–295
3. Bösch P, Nowotny Ch, Schwägerl W, Leber H (1980) Über die Wirkung des Fibrinklebesystems bei orthopädischen Operationen an hämophilen und bei anderen Blutgerinnungsstörungen in: Fibrinogen, Fibrin und Fibrinkleber, Schimpf KL (Hrsg), F K Schattauer Verlag, 275–277
4. Feddersen C (1980) Application of the fibrinogen adhesive method for the definitive hemostasis of posttraumatic repeated bleeding episodes in a boy with hemophilia-A inhibitor. Hämophilie-symp Hamburg 1978, Landbeck G, Marx R (Hrsg), Global Druck u. Verlag, Heidelberg 185–194
5. Feddersen C (1983) The fibrin adhesion system employed for definitive haemostasis and healing in a haemophilia-A inhibitor patient. Scient. Workshop Aarhus 1982, Skjol Dborg H (Hrsg), Immuno Wien, 59–63
6. Puhl W, Böhm B, Schimpf KL, Braun A (1982) Fibrin zur Blutstillung am spongiösen Knochen bei Hämophilie in: Fibrinkleber in Orthopädie und Traumatologie. Cotta H, Braun A (Hrsg), Georg Thieme Verlag Stuttgart, 88–90
7. Torri G, Ventura R, Peretti G, Pietrogrande V (1979) L'uso della colla di fibrina nella chirurgia dell'emofilico. Atti e memorie della Sotimi 37, 1–6
8. Torri G, Lozey E, Cerea P, Motta F, Bonfiglio G (1982) Terapia chirurgica delle cisti emofiliche: la nostra esperienza nell'empiego del fibrinogeno umano (Tissucol Immuno) Ort e Traum Oggi, Vol II N. 1
9. Torri G, Ventura R, Leonardi M, Marinoni EC (1984) Nostra esperienza sul Tissucol in chirurgia Ortopedica: Chirurgia dell'emofilico, chirurgia nervosa, chirurgia dei tendini ed innesti osteocartilaginei. Clot Hematol. Malignancies 1, 31–34

The Use of Fibrin Sealant in Orthopaedic Surgery of Coagulation Diseases, with Special Reference to Haemophilic Cysts and Pseudotumours

F. Fernandez-Palazzi, S. Rivas Hernandez, and M. Rupcich

Key words: Surgery coagulation diseases, haemophilic cysts

Abstract

A preliminary report is made on the use of fibrin sealant as an adjunct in cases of coagulation diseases requiring surgery. After a brief comment on fibrin sealant properties as an antihaemorrhagic, adhesive and binding material, the experience of the Orthopaedic Unit of the National Haemophilia Treatment Center of the Municipal Blood Bank and the Orthopaedic Service "C" of the Hospital San Juan de Dios in Caracas, Venezuela, is presented. The material consists of 14 cases with blood dyscrasia where fibrin sealant was used as an adjunct to surgery. The pathologies were haemophilia A and B, para-haemophilia XIII, disfibrinogenaemia, intravascular disseminated coagulation, activated anti-X factor, lymphoma, and inhibitor factor XIII. A newly developed method of percutaneous treatment of haemophilic cysts and pseudotumours with voidment and refill with fibrin sealant is described.

Introduction

In orthopaedic surgery there are some pathological entities representing a challenge when considering operative procedures, due not only to their surgical difficulty, but to the great morbidity and mortality involved. These are cases of blood dyscrasia, and among them those involving haemophilia.

There have been many advances in the past 2 decades towards solving the problems involved in surgery in these patients, diminishing both morbility and mortality; it is now possible to perform surgery that was unbelievable some years ago. The main advance was the possibility of obtaining the deficient factors for coverage (VIII, IX, XIII, fibrinogen, etc.), making it possible to raise the deficient factor to a normal level, thus transforming surgery in these patients in a procedure similar to that known in general orthopaedics. Nevertheless, there are still the problems of excessive bleeding during surgery and difficulty in obtaining a good seal of empty spaces and skin sutures.

The purpose of this paper is to give a preliminary report on the use of fibrin sealant in orthopaedic surgery of blood dyscrasia.

Fibrin Sealant in Operative Medicine
Traumatology and Orthopaedics – Vol. 7
Edited by G. Schlag, H. Redl
© Springer-Verlag Berlin Heidelberg 1986

Fibrin Sealant

The use of a combination of coagulant substances to produce haemostasis and help wound closure was first made by Gray and Harvey in 1915–1916 [6], utilizing a fibrin tampon to control bleeding. This method, in spite of not being completely success-ful, initiated a series of studies and development of new procedures and materials. In the decade of the 1970s Immuno, Austria, developed a method of cryoprecipita-tion, to obtain highly concentrated fibrinogen solutions, with a high content of factor XIII. This method made it possible to revive the system of sealing by means of fibrin coagulum, and its successful application [2, 3, 4, 6, 7, 8, 9].

This material was first used at the Traumatology Center of the Lorenz Bohler Hospital in Vienna by Matras and Kuderna in 1973, on suturing median and ulnar nerves by means of fibrin sealant [5].

Biochemistry and Action of Fibrin Sealant

The commercial preparation named Tissucol/Tisseel (Immuno AG) consists of two different components:
1. Fibrinogen: factor XIII in a high concentration, plus some other plasmatic proteins such as albumin and globulin, not soluble at low temperatures; these are the active factors of the preparation. Aprotinin as an inhibitor of fibrinolysis.
2. A solution of thrombin and calcium chloride that precipitates the above-men-tioned component.

The mixture of these two components starts the coagulation process, the seal solidifies and the resulting coagulum is stabilized due to the union through fibrin. The two components must be previously mixed, in different proportions according to the speed of coagulation and solidification required. If a rapid response and sealing is desired, 500 U thrombin are necessary. If more time to work is required, thus giving a slower solidification time, 4 U thrombin should be used.

There are three properties of fibrin sealant:
1. Haemostasis: due to coagulant substances such as fibrin, fibrinogen and calcium chloride. The fibrin clot formed lasts for 8–14 days, depending on the fibrinolytic activity of the tissue involved.
2. Sealing: the sealing produced achieves useful solid resistance after 5 min. The optimum mechanical solidity is obtained after 24 h.
3. Cicatrization: the fibrin union produces an ideal matress for fibroblast growing. The synthesis of collagen by the fibroblast leads to fibrous tissue proliferation and the cicatrization of the wound.

Material

Since 1981 we have used fibrin sealant in the Orthopaedic Unit of the National Haemophilia Treatment Center of the Municipal Blood Bank and at the Orthopaedic Service C of the Hospital San Juan de Dios in Caracas, Venezuela.

According to the blood dyscrasia the patients were grouped:

Haemophilia VIII	7 cases
Haemophilia IX	1 case
Parahaemophilia XIII	2 cases
Disfibrinogenaemia	1 case
Intravascular disseminated coagulation	1 case
Activated anti-X factor + lymphoma	1 case
Inhibitor factor VIII (40 Bethesda units)	1 case

Indications for fibrin sealant:

Haematoma Thigh	1 case
Zygoma	1 case
Biopsy Neck lymph node	1 case
Mediastinum	1 case
Lung	1 case
Finger wound	1 case
Skin necrosis	1 case
Pseudotumours Tibia	1 case
Foot	1 case
Iliacus	1 case
Cysts Humerus	2 cases
Isquium	1 case
Nasal bleeding	1 case

1. T.C., male, age 78 years. Absence of factor XIII. Post-traumatic haematoma in the left thigh, drained through three incisions. Acute peroperatory haemorrhage, required fibrinogen 9.5 g, fresh blood 12 U, globular concentrate 5 U, platelet concentrate 6 U, Capramol 2.5 g, fresh plasma 9 U and antihaemophilic factor 5000 U.
   For stopping bleeding the treatment required three different sittings every 2nd day and a total of 23 ml fibrin sealant. Patient died of peritonitis in January 1981.

2. J.C.U., male, age 10 years. Absence of factor XIII. Biopsy and removal of neck lymph node. One millilitre fibrin sealant was used as haemostatic and for wound closure. Pathology reported chronic adenitis. Healing satisfactory April 1981.

3. F.V., male, age 74 years. Disfibrinogenaemia, probable Hodkins. A mediastinum biopsy was performed. There was some parenchymatous bleeding, controlled with 1 ml fibrin sealant. Muscular bleeding subsided with 1 ml fibrin sealant in January 1981.

4. G.C., male, age 19 years. Haemophilia A, factor VIII higher than 5%. Post-traumatic haematoma in left cheek bone (encapsulated). Surgical resection. Haemostasia and skin suture with 1 ml fibrin sealant. September 1981.

5. M.V., female age 49 years. Intravascular disseminated coagulation, post general surgery, with pulmonary insufficiency. A lung biopsy was performed. Pathology confirmed diagnosis of peumonitis. Parenchymatous bleeding was controlled with 2 ml fibrin sealant. October 1981.

6. M.S., male, age 12 years. Severe haemophilia A with inhibitors. Clean cut wound fourth finger right hand, closed using only 1 ml fibrin sealant. December 1981.

7. I.J., female, age 43 years. Activated anti-X factor, multiple lymphoma. Necrosis skin flexor face of forearm post 131 I injection. A necrectomy was performed and a free skin graft done for coverage; 4 ml fibrin sealant was used to attach skin graft after haemostasia carried out. March 1982.

8. S.R., male, age 10 years. Mild haemophilia B. Pseudotumor right lower tibia lasting 3 years. A surgical resection plus musculocutaneous skin graft was performed in two stages. First, a curetage resection of the pseudotumour filled with homologous preserved graft (Kiel) using 4 ml fibrin sealant to assist gluing the graft. A gastrognemious musculocutaneous flap was performed on left leg and sutured to the gap remaining from the resection and after an Achilles tendon lengthening; 2 ml fibrin sealant was used as haemostatic in the flap. A free skin graft covered the donor site and 2 ml fibrin sealant was used. The second stage took place 3 weeks later in order to detach the flap, requiring 2 ml fibrin sealant as a haemostatic and a further 2 ml when suturing. The result was very satisfactory, with the patient able to walk with crutches 1 month after surgery, after being 3 years in bed. March 1982 [1].

9. J.C.T., male, age 10 years. Mild haemphilia A. Pseudotumor right foot compromising tarsal and metatarsal bones, first seen at the clinic after 6 months of development. Due to its size, debridements (removal of necrotic bone and soft tissue slough) were performed every 2 day, under factor VIII cover; local cures were finished every time packing with antibiotic pomade (Gentalyn) plus Gelfoam. The size was so reduced that a secondary cicatrization of the defect was made, helped by 1 ml fibrin sealant (Fig. 1). The final result was quite satisfactory but some equinus due to shortening of Achilles tendon was present caused by the long periods of immobility. January 1985.

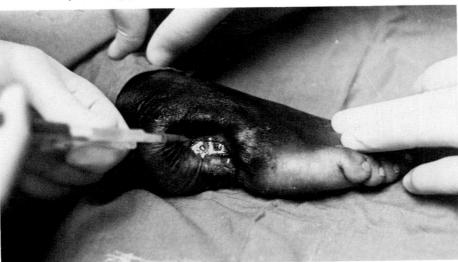

Fig. 1. Case 9: Pseudotumor in the right foot. Secondary cicatrization of the defect enforced with fibrin sealant

10. G.L., female, age 65 years, with idiopathic lung fibrosis, developed sudden nasal bleeding. An inhibitor factor VIII (40 Bethesda units) was present; it was impossible to stop the bleeding in spite of cover with 7500 U factor VIII and ligature of corresponding nasal artery. The bleeding stopped after performing a nasal packing with 2 ml fibrin sealant. November 1984.

Percutaneous Treatment of Haemophilic Cysts and Pseudotumours

This pathology, first reported by Starker in 1918 [3], can be described as an encapsulated reservoir of blood with a tendency to grow and increase in size, either slowly or rapidly, and, depending on its location can invade neighbouring tissue, imitating a neoformation or a tumor. It is a characteristic pathology of haemophiliacs, appearing more frequently between 1nd and 3rd decades of life. This formation is called cyst when small and with little trabeculation, and pseudotumor when big, lobulated and invasive.

According to its etiology it can be spontaneous with no cause for bleeding in a close space, and post-traumatic, when an external trauma is the cause of the bleeding.

According to its origin it is named "true" when caused by intraosseous bleeding and "false" when originating from encapsulated muscular haematomas, located in muscles with strong fascial coverage, or from gross tendinous or large muscle insertion.

According to its location the cyst can be present in soft tissue, subperiostical or juxta-articular osseous tissue, and intraosseous tissue. It appears more frequently in the femur than in the pelvis, followed by the tibia, foot, hand, humerus, mandible and radius. The location depends on bone maturity; for this reason in children this lesion appears more frequently distally (forearm, leg, hand and foot) and in adults it is usually seen in proximal locations (pelvis, femoral and humeral epiphysis).

Clinically the increase in size is not always accompanied by pain. In rapidly growing cysts there is pain, together with elastic consistency and expansive agressivity. Intraosseous cysts are originally hard but become elastic when destroying the cortex in the growing process.

The radiological aspect of these cysts and pseudotumors is not characteristic; on the contrary, it can be confusing, making differential diagnosis from real neoplasia difficult. Those cysts located in soft tissues are seen in X-rays as dense areas with diffused borders, overlapping neighbouring tissues. Those which are subperiostical or juxta-articular osseous are seen as enlarged or periostical elevations and the bone cortex can show signs of compression. Those which are intraosseous or true cysts are shown as trabeculated or lobulated osteolytic areas, and, as they grow, can destroy the bone cortex.

Since November 1982 we have developed a new method of percutaneous treatment for early haemophilic cysts and advanced pseudotumours which are non-surgically resectable. In these cases we proceed with an X-ray image amplifier to locate the lesion, percutaneously introducing a large trocar until reaching the cyst (Fig. 2). Through this trocar the lesion is emptied of all its contents, mostly pure blood. Under pressure the space is filled with fibrin sealant and the trocar removed.

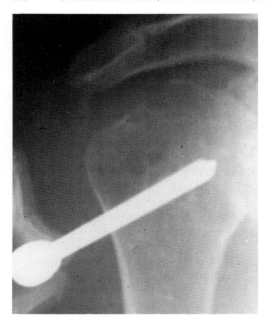

Fig. 2. Introduction of the trocar into the cyst under an X-ray image amplifier

The amount of fibrin sealant to be used varies according to the size of the cysts, requiring 1 ml fibrin sealant to cover or spread a space of 4 cm^2, that is a proportion of 1 to 4. Thus, for a lesion of approximately 8 cm^2 we use 2 ml fibrin sealant, which is presented in the Tissucol Kit 2, and for a 40 cm^2 lesion quantity of 10 ml fibrin sealant is required.

The main advantages of this treatment are the easy technique, the lack of agressivity, by being percutaneous a requirement for very little coverage with antihaemophilic factor, and an ability sometimes to be performed on ambulatory bases, thus lowering the cost of the treatment. In non-surgically resectable pseudotumours this procedure seems to stop the progression of the lesion.

11. F.G., male age 18 years. Haemophilia A, with 5% factor VIII. Presented pain and limitation of movement of right shoulder for 6 months. X-rays and CT scan demonstrated a cyst on proximal right humerus. In the procedure 6 ml blood was aspirated and the cyst filled with 2 ml fibrin sealant (Fig. 3). After 7 days hospitalization and couverage with 36 680 U factor VIII, the shoulder was painless and normal range of motion was recovered after 1 month. After 2 months X-rays proved the disappearance of the cyst. November 1982.

12. M.L., male, age 22 years. Haemophilia A with 5.5% factor VIII. After having pain in the scapular region and shoulder for 1 year, diminution of shoulder abduction (60%) and severe muscular atrophy were seen. X-rays showed a cyst on proximal left humerus. In the procedure 11 ml blood was aspirated and the lesion filled with 2 ml fibrin sealant. The factor VIII coverage was 5750 U and the patient stayed in hospital for 2 days, was painless after 1 month, and abduction recovered up to 80° after 6 months. After 2 months the cyst disappeared in X-ray image. January 1984.

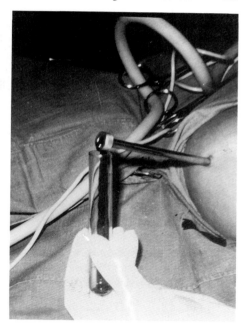

Fig. 3. Case 11: percutaneous aspiration of the blood in the cyst

13. M.S., male, age 13 years. Haemophilia A with 1.1% factor VIII, inhibitors 2.5 Bethesda units. Complained of pain at left isquium for 15 days, with irradiation to left thigh, interfering with walking. X-ray showed cyst in left isquium. In the procedure 5 ml blood was aspirated and the cysts filled with 1 ml fibrin sealant. Total coverage of factor VIII was 15 640 U and hospitalization time was 3 days. There was total disappearance of pain after 1 week with recovery of normal range of movement and ability to walk. June 1984.

In these three cases of small cysts we used fast-solidyfing fibrin sealant, adding 500 U thrombin on preparation.

14. F.L., male, age 37 years. Haemophilia A with 1% factor VIII and inhibitors reported previously but not at the time of surgery. When seen the patient presented pseudotumour in left iliac region developed from a psoas haematoma not treated and growing slowly for 4 years. Complained of pain, functional impairment and increased volume of involved area. The pseudotumor had invaded left iliac crest, which had almost completely disappeared, and acetabular roof, isquium and surrounding soft tissues down to trochanteric region. Due to his severe haemophilia requiring repetitive coverage with factor VIII, he presented kidney and liver problems. Any kind of surgical removal was considered very dangerous "quo ad vitam". Thus we intended this procedure to stop progression. In November 1984 we emptied the lesion through three approaches: two above and one below iliac crest (Fig. 4); 1000 ml blood was obtained by aspiration. The case required 10 ml fibrin sealant (6 ml slow solidification to cover the wall and 4 ml fast solidification to fix the above);

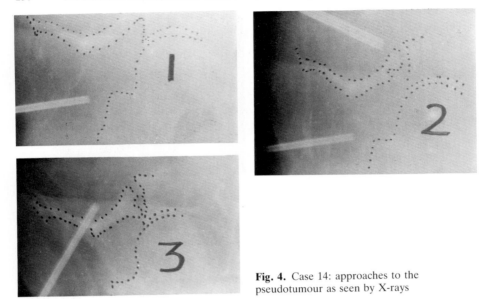

Fig. 4. Case 14: approaches to the pseudotumour as seen by X-rays

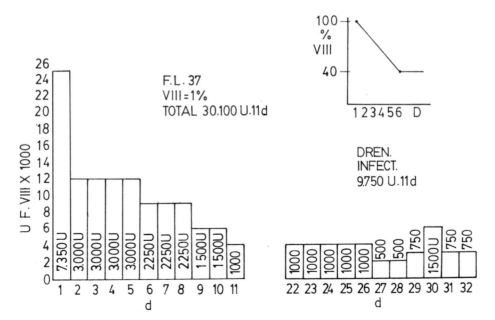

Fig. 5. Case 15: coverage and levels obtained of factor VIII

30 000 U factor VIII was required and time of hospitalization was 11 days. There was evident diminution of size of tumor and most of the pain disappeared, the discomfort remaining due to its location. The range of movement improved slightly but he was able to walk with crutches. X-rays showed reduction of size after 2 months. A local infection in one puncture site developed after 22 days, requiring drainage and 9750 U antihaemophilic factor (Fig. 5). Three months after the procedure the patient developed terminal kidney failure requiring haemodialysis. Died from AIDS 7 months after the operation.

References

1. Carlesso J, Fernández-Palazzi F (1984) Uso del colgajo miocutaneo de pierna cruzada, usando el gastrognemio medialis, en un paciente hemofílico B. Rev Hospital San Juan de Dios 5: 9–10
2. Fernández-Palazzi F, Silva J, Gamarra J (1981) Informe preliminar sobre el uso de la cola de fibrina en cirugía ortopédica. Centro Médico 70: 157–166
3. Fernández-Palazzi F, Rivas S, Rupcich M (1985) Experience with fibrin seal in the management of haemophilic cysts and pseudotumors. Proceedings. Management of Musculosqueletal problems in haemophilia, 22–23 feb 1985 Denver, Colorado
4. Fernández-Palazzi F, Bosch N. Rupcich M, Brínez M (1986) Trattamento dei pseudo-cisti emofilici nell'ospedale San Juan de Dios. Traumatologia Ortopedia Oggi (To be published)
5. Matras M, Inges M, Lassman M, Mammoli B (1973) Non sutures nerve transplantation. J Maxilofac Surg 1: 37
6. Schlag G (1980) Personal communication
7. Schlag G (1981) Hemostasia, sutura y reconstrucción con la Cola de Fibrina (Nuevo Método) Centro Médico 70: 153–156
8. Staindl O (1979) The healing of wounds and scar formation under the influence of a tissue adhesion system with fibrinogen, thrombin and coagulation factor XIII Arch Otorhinolar 222: 241–245
9. Urlesberger K (1979) Fibrin adhesive in surgery of renal parenchyma Em Urol 5: 260–261

Haemostatic Effect of Fibrin Sealant in Patients with Congenital and Acquired Bleeding Disorders

F. BAUDO and F. de CATALDO

Key words: bleeding disorders, tooth extraction, local hemostasis

Abstract

Fibrin sealant was used for local hemostasis in 405 patients with various hemostatic disorders (thrombocytopenia, chronic liver disease, hemophilia A and B, von Willebrand's disease and oral anticoagulants) undergoing tooth extraction. Prophylactic replacement therapy (platelets or plasma concentrates) and antifibrinolytic agents were not administered. Oral anticoagulants were not discontinued. Minor postextraction bleeding occurred only in severe hemophilia A and occasionally in the oral anticoagulant group.

Introduction

Fibrin sealant has been used for its local hemostatic effect in various clinical conditions, in patients with either normal or abnormal hemostasis. Fields of application range widely: cardiac and vascular surgery [1, 2], hepatectomy [3], neurosurgery [4], orthopedic surgery [5], stomatology [6] and otorhinolaryngology [7].

Tooth extraction in patients with hereditary and acquired hemostatic disorders requires specific replacement therapy in order to avoid severe bleeding. It is therefore particularly appropriate to demonstrate the hemostatic effect of this product when locally applied. We shall discuss our experience with 405 patients with various types of bleeding disorders who underwent tooth extraction.

Patients

A total of 405 patients undergoing tooth extraction (for diagnosis and relevant laboratory data, see tables) have been treated. Of these, 150 patients had multiple extractions in the same session. Prophylactic replacement therapy with platelets or plasma concentrates and antifibrinolytic agents was not given. Oral anticoagulants were not discontinued.

Technique

Fibrin sealant was applied into the alveolar cavity that was successively filled with collagen felt (B. Braun AG, Melsungen, FRG) kept in place by suture.

Fibrin Sealant in Operative Medicine
Traumatology and Orthopaedics – Vol. 7
Edited by G. Schlag, H. Redl
© Springer-Verlag Berlin Heidelberg 1986

Results and Comments

Data on patients affected by chronic liver disease and acquired hypoprothrombinemia are given in Table 1. There were 62 extractions in 33 patients, 18 of whom had multiple extractions. The platelet count was $30–90 \times 10^9/l$, and the Normotest values ranged from 18% to 35%. No prophylactic replacement therapy with concentrates (prothrombin complex or/and platelets) was given; no bleeding occurred.

Data on patients affected by thrombocytopenia are given in Table 2. There were 1 case of bone marrow hypoplasia, 6 chronic lymphocytic leukemia, 7 acute nonlymphocytic leukemia, and 4 chronic idiopathic thrombocytopenia. The platelet count was $10–70 \times 10^9/l$. No prophylaxis was given and no bleeding occurred.

Data on patients on oral anticoagulant therapy are in Table 3. There were 319 patients with prosthetic heart valves who had 478 extractions; 108 of them had multiple extractions. In these patients the oral anticoagulant therapy was not discontinued because of the high risk of thromboembolic complications. The

Table 1. Tissucol in tooth extractions in patients with chronic liver disease and thrombocytopenia

Patients	33	
Platelets	$30–90 \times 10^9/l$	($\bar{x}$ 65)
Normotest	18%–35%	($\bar{x}$ 24)
Extractions	62 (1–6/patient)	
Prophylaxis	0	
Bleeding complications	0	

Table 2. Tissucol in tooth extractions in thrombocytopenia

Cases (n)	Diagnosis	Platelets ($\times 10^9/l$)	Extractions	Bleeding complications
1	Bone marrow hypoplasia	20–32	9 (in 4 sessions)	0
6	Chronic lymphocytic leukemia	10–40	16	0
7	Acute non lymphocytic leukemia	15–45	17	0
4	Chronic idiopathic thrombocytopenia	40–70	6	0

Table 3. Tissucol in tooth extractions in patients on oral anticoagulants

Patients	319
Thrombotest	5%–13%
Extractions	478 (1–5/patient)
Bleeding complications	25
Replacement therapy[a]	2

[a] Single infusion of "prothrombin" concentrate 10 u/kg

Table 4. Tissucol in tooth extractions in hemophilia and von Willebrand's disease

Patients (n)	Factor deficiency	u/ml	Extractions	Bleeding complications	Replacement therapy
12	VIII	< 0.01	29	7	7[a]
16[b]	VIII	< 0.10	24	1	0
1	IX	< 0.01	1	0	–
6	vW	< 0.05	7	0	–

vW, von Willebrand
[a] Single infusion of Factor VIII concentrate (15 u/kg)
[b] A patient with chronic liver disease (Normotest 30%, platelets $90 \times 10^9/l$)

therapy was monitored by the Thrombotest mantained in the therapeutic range (5%–13%). While 25 patients had bleeding, only two required replacement therapy: a single infusion of prothrombincomplex concentrate (10 u/kg). In the remaining 23 patients bleeding ceased after the stitches were removed.

Data on hereditary bleeding disorders (hemophilia and von Willebrand's disease) are in Table 4. These were 12 cases of severe hemophilia A (factor VIII: C < 1%), 16 mild hemophilia A (Factor VIII: C < 10%), 1 severe hemophilia B (Factor IX: C < 1%), 6 von Willebrand (bleeding time > 20'). Bleeding occurred in 7 severe hemophiliacs 24–48 h after extraction and was controlled by removal of the stitches and low dose replacement therapy (single infusion of 15 u/kg of Factor VIII concentrate). Tooth extraction was uneventful in mild hemophilia and von Willebrand patients.

Tooth extraction in these clinical settings is a remarkable challange to the hemostatic mechanism. These data substantiate the efficacy of Tissucol in controlling traumatic bleeding when hemostasis is impaired.

References

1. Borst HG, Haverich A, Walterbusch G, Maatz W (1982) Fibrin adhesive: an important hemostatic adjunct in cardiovascular operations. Thorac J Cardiovasc Surg 84: 548–553
2. Eckersberger F, Holle J, Wolner E, Navratil J, Lindner A (1980) Fibrin adhesive human-liquid and fibrin adhesive human lyophilized for hemostasis in open heart surgery. In: Fibrinogen, Fibrin und Fibrinkleber. Schimpf Kl (Hrsg). Schattauer FK Verlag, 257
3. Spängler HP (1980) Erfahrungen mit Fibrin zur Gewebeklebung, und lokalen Blutstillung in der Abdominalchirurgie. In: Fibrinogen, Fibrin und Fibrinkleber, Schimpf Kl (Hrsg). Schattauer FKVerlag, 263–264
4. Haase J Fibrin sealing in a case of intractable bleeding from a glioblastoma. Scient. Workshop Aarhus, 1982 H. Skjoidborg (Hrsg), Immuno Wien: 95–96
5. Bösh P, Nowotny Ch, Schwägerl W, Leber H (1982) Über die Wirkung des Fibrinklebesystems bei orthopädischen Operationen an Hämophilen und bei anderen Blutgerinnungsstörungen. In: Fibrinogen, Fibrin und Fibrinkleber; Schimpf KL (Hrsg). Schattauer FK, Verlag, 275–277
6. Wepner F, Fries R, Platz H (1982) The use of the fibrin adhesive system for local hemostasis in oral surgery. Oral J maxillofac. Surg 40: 555–558
7. Gastpar H (1979) Erfahrungen mit einem humanen Fibrinkleber bei operativen Eingriffen im Kopf-Hals-Bereich. Laryng Rhinol otol 58: 389–399

Subject Index